P9-CEZ-495

WORK IT OUT

A Mood-Boosting Exercise Guide for
People Who Just Want to Lie Down

SARAH KURCHAK

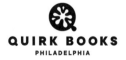

QUIRK BOOKS

PHILADELPHIA

Copyright © 2023 by Quirk Productions, Inc.

All rights reserved. Except as authorized under U.S. copyright law, no part of this book may be reproduced in any form without written permission from the publisher.

Library of Congress Cataloging-in-Publication Data

Names: Kurchak, Sarah, 1982- author.

Title: Work it out : a mood-boosting exercise guide for people who just want to lie down / Sarah Kurchak.

Description: Philadelphia, PA : Quirk Books, [2023] | Summary: "A guide to incorporating exercise into daily life to improve mental health. The book dispels fitness myths and provides practical advice for building adjustable workout plans, celebrating even minor achievements, and knowing when to rest"— Provided by publisher.

Identifiers: LCCN 2022038847 (print) | LCCN 2022038848 (ebook) | ISBN 9781683693291 (paperback) | ISBN 9781683693307 (ebook)

Subjects: LCSH: Exercise—Psychological aspects. | Physical fitness—Psychological aspects. | Mental health promotion. | Mind and body. | Motivation (Psychology)

Classification: LCC GV481.2 .K87 2023 (print) | LCC GV481.2 (ebook) | DDC 613.7/1019—dc23/eng/20220921

LC record available at https://lccn.loc.gov/2022038847

LC ebook record available at https://lccn.loc.gov/2022038848

ISBN: 978-1-68369-329-1

Printed in China

Typeset in Tomarik, Providence Sans, Dreaming Outloud, Freight Text and Freight Sans

Designed by Elissa Flanigan

Production management by John J. McGurk

Quirk Books

215 Church Street

Philadelphia, PA 19106

quirkbooks.com

10 9 8 7 6 5 4 3 2 1

TO MY CLIENTS,
THE LADIES OF THE B AND R,
AND MY YSFC REGULARS

CONTENTS

INTRODUCTION

"Have you tried exercise?"

If you've ever had less than 100 percent perfect mental health, there is a very good chance that some well-meaning person has said this to you. There's an even better chance that some smug and not so well-meaning types have said it, too.

I'm going to take a wild guess and assume that this terribly helpful advice did not fix you.

The problem isn't exercise. It is true, unfortunately, that any physical activity done with any regularity has the potential to improve your mood. It's not a miracle cure or an all-purpose substitute for other interventions—you should not, under any circumstances, drop everything else you've been doing to take care of yourself and give me twenty. But exercise can provide focus, routine, comfort, and even a boost to physical health when it feels like everything else is going to hell. And yes, it can make you feel less like shit.

During the ten years I worked in the fitness industry, I saw a number of clients who had depression and anxiety, and I witnessed the positive influence that our workouts had on their lives. I've also felt the mental benefits of physical movement for myself. I'm not a fan of big, sweeping statements about the power of fitness. I find that kind of overly plucky talk grating and alienating. But it's fair to say that discovering workouts that I enjoyed and regularly doing them has played a part in keeping me alive. And I'm not talking about their effect on my cardiovascular system.

Exercise can help people who are dealing with anxiety and depression. But *telling* them that exercise can help? That's one of the most useless things in the history of fitness. And the history of fitness has given us homeopathic sports supplements, ab-toning belts, magic seaweed yoga pants, and kettle-bell routines for stationary bikes.

"Have you tried exercise?" (or, perhaps even more inescapable, "Have you tried yoga?") is annoying and insulting. Of course you've tried exercise! It's not new. Its ability to boost mental well-being was not obscure or privileged information that had never been imparted to you before some rando decided that the best response to your struggles was, in essence, "Bummer, try jogging that off."

It also completely fails to understand the crux of the issue. Most people who are dealing with conditions like anxiety and depression are already aware—often too aware—of the things we could or should be doing to make our lives better or more manageable. But knowing what you should do, or even what you want to do, and not being able to do it is kind of a big part of the whole being anxious and depressed thing.

When I started researching the topic for my clients and myself, I noticed that most of the accessible articles and information involving exercise and mental health fell into that same trap. The fitness industry is filled with life-hacks for depression, but most of it seems to be coming from a place of ignorance about the cold war going on in the average depressed person's head. The introductions talk about how great exercise is for you, and then they jump straight to tips on motivation, routine, and the physical activity itself. Those tips aren't necessarily wrong, but when you're suffering, they're not realistic.

Moving our bodies within their capabilities is a fundamental part of life. It can be a source of physical and mental well-being. It should be a source of joy.

But so much of the information about how you can do it and the venues to do it in is patrolled by a culture that prefers competition, punishment, and shame. There's clearly a huge need for exercise research, programming, and resources that understand depression. But there's also a need for resources that appreciate how alienated so many people feel from fitness culture—and, indeed, from their own bodies as a result of fitness culture. And there's a desperate need for people with any authority in that realm to acknowledge how hard it is for so many of us to just try exercise, especially when people are already working so hard to stay alive.

With this book, I have an opportunity to do my small part to answer those needs. I've included practical tips for how to find physical activities that you don't hate, how to integrate them into your life, and how to do them safely. I also talk about how and why exercise can help you, how and why it often ends up hurting you instead, and what you can do to try to break that cycle. And I've woven a bunch of validation and encouragement throughout. If you've ever needed an outside source to confirm that getting into exercise isn't easy, that the fitness industry is kind of full of it, and that you're doing your best, it's all there for you. From a former fitness professional, no less, if that helps you take it to heart or gets some judgmental dick off your case.

I've written with a focus on people with depression and anxiety, because that's what I have the most experience with and that's the population I feel most assured addressing directly. But I believe there is plenty of material here that can be useful to any neurodivergent person. Or anyone who is just a little sad, for that matter.

My goal is to help you feel better, so I've eliminated the aspects of fitness that only make people feel worse. There's nothing about diets in here. On a professional level, I'm unqualified to give advice. On a personal note, I hate them. There's definitely nothing about weight loss. The only time I'll discuss weight at all is to acknowledge how abusive and unscientific fatphobia is.

There are other absences from the book that are less righteous, though. The big one, for me, is modifications. I am a huge fan, and I discuss them in a general sense. I encourage you to adapt exercise moves to meet your body's needs instead of the other way around. I remind you that modifying exercises is not cheating and even so-called easy versions can offer new challenges and results. But I don't have the space to include every adaptation for every ability level and for every disability that the trainer in me would love to. You'll have to bring awareness to what your body can and can't do—but what you have from me is blanket permission to skip anything that feels bad in a way that never winds up feeling good. (Or to skip exercise entirely, if its negative effect on your body is worse than its positive effect on your mind. For instance, exercise may be harmful for people with injuries or chronic conditions. If that's you, check in with your body and your doctor before listening to some book!)

Space and scope also limit how geeky I can get about workout plans. I do share basic training ideas and exercises for strength, cardio, and mind-body work, but I don't provide detailed routines. However, I do offer guidance on how to develop your own plans from a menu of options (see the chart on pages 10–11). If you're depressed and looking for tips on how to get into exercising *and* find the perfect workout for developing stability and mobility in the shoulder girdle, for example, this isn't the only resource you'll need. Consider it the warm-up portion of your journey.

If a lot of words are beneficial to your learning and processing styles and you have the mental energy to tackle a whole book, or a whole chapter, you can read this book straight through like you would any other book. If you're running low on energy but could use some suggestions and maybe use a non-perky pep talk or two, you can scan through to find the sidebars and infographics. And if you just want someone to tell you what to do, follow the charts.

And however you use this book, please take the information that works for you and discard the rest. I'm here to help, not dictate. (Although if you would rather be told exactly what to do, there's something here for you, too.) The last thing you need is one more a-hole telling you what you should do.

HOW TO USE THIS BOOK:
WHAT ARE YOU LOOKING FOR TODAY?

TELL ME WHAT TO DO.

WHAT ARE YOU MOST INTERESTED IN RIGHT NOW?

STRENGTH

"HEAVY STUFF," P. 125

CARDIO

"RUN FROM YOUR PROBLEMS," P. 155

MIND/BODY OR FLEXIBILITY

"AROUND THE BEND," P. 99

STILL TOO MUCH THOUGHT. TELL ME EXACTLY WHAT TO DO.

THE F-IT WORKOUT, P. 56

I DON'T WANT TO DO ANYTHING.

DO YOU THINK YOU'LL FEEL BETTER IF YOU DO SOMETHING, EVEN IF YOU DON'T FEEL LIKE IT?

UGH, YES

NOT REALLY

YOU DON'T HAVE TO EXERCISE

I WISH. BUT A PERSON, CIRCUMSTANCE, OR SELF-ESTEEM ISSUE IS PUSHING ME.

OK. TODAY YOU'RE DOING A REST WORKOUT. READ "THROWING IN THE TOWEL," P. 175.

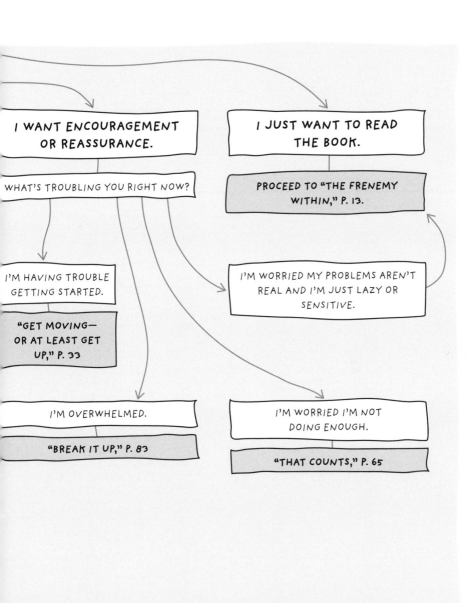

I WANT ENCOURAGEMENT OR REASSURANCE.

I JUST WANT TO READ THE BOOK.

WHAT'S TROUBLING YOU RIGHT NOW?

PROCEED TO "THE FRENEMY WITHIN," P. 13.

I'M HAVING TROUBLE GETTING STARTED.

I'M WORRIED MY PROBLEMS AREN'T REAL AND I'M JUST LAZY OR SENSITIVE.

"GET MOVING—OR AT LEAST GET UP," P. 33

I'M OVERWHELMED.

I'M WORRIED I'M NOT DOING ENOUGH.

"BREAK IT UP," P. 83

"THAT COUNTS," P. 65

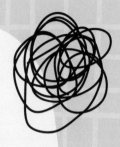

ONE

THE FRENEMY WITHIN

Why exercise is good for your brain—and why your brain is being a pain in the ass about it

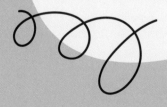

Unfortunately, perky fitness types are right about one thing. Their delivery sucks and they tend to overstate the case, but they're not wrong about this: exercise can help reduce anxiety and depression symptoms. (The *can* and the *help* are doing some lifting here, but they're not lifting heavy.)

If you engage in a moderate amount of physical activity on a fairly regular basis, there is a good chance that it will noticeably improve your mood. If you have anxiety or depression, it might also prevent some of your symptoms from coming back if and when you're feeling better. Exercise doesn't work this way for everyone, and it's not a cure for mental illness. It also can't fix many of the circumstances that might be contributing to your issues. You can't burpee your way out of late-stage capitalism or outrun climate change. But the odds are good that consistent movement can take some of the edge off of what you're going through.

How does this work? The short answer is that we don't exactly know yet. Studies on the subject consistently find that exercise has a measurable positive influence on mental well-being, but we need more research to know what makes that happen. Anxiety and depression are complex, and our understanding of the brain is constantly evolving and far from complete. Meanwhile, our understanding of exercise is going through its own growing pains.

There are some predominating theories, though.

WE DON'T KNOW WHY EXERCISE HELPS, BUT WE HAVE SOME GUESSES

The theory that you're most likely to encounter in fitness circles involves endorphins. These neurotransmitters, or natural brain chemicals, are released during enjoyable activities like laughing and sex to increase your pleasure. In less fun moments, such as suffering an injury, your body will also produce a rush of endorphins to temporarily alleviate discomfort and stress. So the idea is that exercise stimulates the release of endorphins that, in turn, can reduce stress and anxiety, improve your self-esteem, and boost your overall mood. The runner's high—the phenomenon in which a person experiences a sudden rush of euphoria in the middle of an otherwise un-euphoric run—is an example of this. Endorphins can also contribute to your general well-being by reducing pain and inflammation.

While endorphins get the bulk of the attention in Depression and Exercise 101 messaging, though, they're not the only neurotransmitter that might be involved. Another hypothesis revolves around dopamine, serotonin, and norepinephrine. Dopamine plays a major role in how we experience pleasure and helps regulate executive function, memory, mood, sleep, and stress. Serotonin is a mood stabilizer that can reduce symptoms of depression and anxiety. Norepinephrine is instrumental in the fight-or-flight response and can help with concentration and overall mood. People experiencing depression often have low levels of all three. Movement encourages neurotransmitter development, so proponents of this theory believe that exercise can help make up the deficit. (At least, that's how we think neurotransmitters work. The human brain is incredibly complex, and all of this is still a work in progress. We're still figuring it out, and probably always will be.)

Other experts believe the connection between exercise and mental health might have more to do with the structure of the brain. Scientists have observed that some people with recurring depression have a smaller hippocampus, which is the part of the brain that deals with mood regulation. This theory suggests that exercise encourages new nerve cell growth and connections in the area, which could lead to more stable moods. Or maybe it comes down to body heat. Elevating your core temperature through exercise reduces muscle tension and improves brain function. There's another theory that suggests this could lead to a reduction in depression and anxiety symptoms.

Then we get into the potential psychological explanations. Exercise can give you a sense of accomplishment and self-efficacy. Depression and burnout often make you feel worthless and like nothing is possible. Every move you execute, every workout you complete, and every goal you reach chips away at that lie. This gives your confidence a much-needed boost and helps you identify a connection between effort and positive outcomes. Exercise can be a decent coping mechanism or a useful distraction from what is troubling you. Depending on the type you choose, it might also open up new social opportunities and help you develop a sense of community. Any one or more of these could contribute to a better headspace.

Some experts believe that seeing physical changes in your body can contribute to this headspace, too. I don't entirely disagree, but I think this theory needs to be approached with nuance and caution.

Our bodies do all sorts of amazing things in response to movement, but our society only celebrates a narrow range of those developments in a narrow range of bodies. Your feelings about changes that occur in your body as the result of exercise—even if they fall within that range—are likely to be influenced by how the world treats you and how you treat yourself as a result of living in that society. Seeing gains and taking pride in them can have a positive impact on your mental well-being, but changing your shape and how you feel about it can be a mixed bag.

It's also entirely possible that none of the above is the one true explanation for the relationship between exercise and mental health. It could be some combination of neuroscience, biology, psychology, and social factors. Or something else entirely. The truth is that our understanding of the subject isn't much more sophisticated than the Insane Clown Posse's grasp of magnets. Fortunately, we don't need to know precisely how exercise operates on the brain and why it might boost our moods to experience this benefit.

What we do know, with as much certainty as is possible in this area of study, is that regular movement has the potential to positively influence your mental well-being. And that movement doesn't have to be particularly demanding or time-consuming. As little as 10 to 15 minutes of moderate effort at a time can make a difference. Some experts believe more intense and longer exercise might make you feel better faster, but we don't know that for sure, either. Even if that theory is true, consistency appears to be the most important factor. Ten to 15 minutes of an activity that you enjoy—or at least tolerate—and can do multiple times a week for a number of weeks is going to do a hell of a lot more for you than 30 minutes of something unpleasant or potentially dangerous that you're going to struggle to keep up for any length of time.

There's no evidence that your brain cares what *kind* of exercise you do. Studies that compare cardio and strength-based workouts have found that they tend to lead to similar results. Your exercise of choice doesn't even have to be anything that we traditionally consider exercise. Plenty of research shows that regular physical activity can improve your mood. And physical activity encompasses everything from walking to housework and gardening to wandering around your home and flailing your limbs in abject despair.

Basically, if you move your body in ways that work for you and you keep doing it, there is a good chance that you will start to feel less crappy.

Just because it sounds simple on paper doesn't mean it's easy, though. If it were, you wouldn't be reading this book, and in fact this book wouldn't need to exist.

WHY WON'T YOUR
BRAIN LET YOU HELP IT?

There are many factors that can mess with your efforts to start and maintain a fitness routine. And one of the main reasons it's hard to stay active? Your brain! Yes, in a particularly cruel irony, all those little-understood processes that you want to help with exercise can thwart your efforts to exercise in the first place. Low dopamine can make you apathetic and exhausted. People with atypical depression (*atypical* here means that it may not look like the textbook definition of depression, not that this type of depression is uncommon) might also have something called *leaden paralysis*, which makes your limbs feel heavy and almost impossible to move. Depression can also mess with your sleeping habits and appetite, which will further drain your energy and motivation. And then it goes and tells you that suck, you're lazy, and nothing you try ever works out anyway.

Anxiety can express itself in so many counterproductive ways. Your body's response to physical exertion might feel exactly like the symptoms of a panic attack. This can be helpful for some people. Sometimes I'm able to head off the worst of an episode with sprints; knowing why my heart rate is elevated and feeling somewhat in control of it grounds me. But for others, feeling those all-too-familiar symptoms exacerbates their problems and makes exercise confusing and unpleasant at best, intolerable at worst. Anxiety related to social situations, health, injury risk, pain, and unfamiliar physical sensations can also hamper your desire and ability to work out.

Other types of neurodivergence come with their own challenges. ADHDers might struggle to find exercise that provides the right kind of stimulation to keep them motivated and focused. Starting new things and transitioning between activities and modes are rarely among autistic people's favorite activities. (It takes me a lot of time and mental energy to prepare for a workout and start it. It takes an equal amount for me to return to the rest of my day when

I'm done.) Sensory sensitivities and coordination issues could be concerns for both groups. Some of us also have a tendency to set unrealistic goals for ourselves, which means we run the risk of jumping into workouts before we're ready for them and hurting our body, our fragile self-confidence, and any desire we might have to try again in the future.

And you don't have to have a diagnosis to have brain stuff that makes it challenging to exercise. You don't need a name for what you're going through—or any idea at all what's up at all, really. A case of trying to survive in this world is more than enough to leave you down, overwhelmed, and burned out.

Of course, your brain and your body are inseparable, and sometimes physical health gets in the way of using exercise to improve your mood. If you have physical health issues, there's a chance you'll need to find exercises and modifications suited to your needs—which can add even more to your mental load, as you need to spend time learning what works for you and making sure that you perform it with the necessary amount of care.

There is also a possibility that you might have to severely alter your workouts or skip them entirely. Our society loves to talk about exercise like it's a universally good thing, but the reality is more complicated. For example, exercise can make the chronic illness myalgic encephalomyelitis/chronic fatigue syndrome (ME/CFS) worse. This is usually the part where a fitness professional would trot out our classic "Consult with a doctor before starting any exercise program" line. I do recommend that, but I've also worked with and cared about enough people who have chronic illnesses to know that not everyone has access to medical experts who are knowledgeable and compassionate enough about these issues to provide you the best advice and care. So I'm also going to recommend seeking the wisdom and support of ME/CFS and chronic illness communities.

Getting into exercise only becomes more complicated, daunting, and tiring when you're dealing with any combination of the above, which many of us are. Basically, we're like video-game characters whose health monitors have almost run out, and the only way to power up is to keep doing the things that are harder to do because our health monitors have already run out. And the soundtrack to this game is an almost constant stream of negative self-talk.

OUTSIDE INFLUENCES MAKE IT WAY HARDER, AND OUTSIDE INFLUENCES ARE FUCKED UP

But our bodies and minds are not the problem here—even if, yes, sometimes they resist our efforts to do the very thing we know they need to feel better. In a vacuum, I believe that we'd be able to find exercises that address our needs and enrich our lives without undue frustration and pain. We're not doing any of this in anything close to a neutral climate, though. We live in a deeply flawed culture that bombards us with harmful messages about work ethic, bodies, and health. Almost everything we can do to genuinely take better care of ourselves is gatekept by industries that exploit those messages for their own gain. And we have to navigate this toxic slurry while carrying around an enormous amount of baggage—if not outright trauma—from our past experiences with it.

There's just no question that our society is rotten with racism, sexism, classism, ableism, and fatphobia, and from the moment we're born into it, we're told lies about ourselves and each other. Some of those lies:

- Hard work is inherently good. Even if (maybe especially if) it hurts you.

- Rest is lazy and therefore bad.

- There is such a thing as a perfect body, and the standards for this perfection are extremely narrow, but everyone can achieve it if they work hard enough.

- There's also such a thing as perfect health and it's equally possible for everyone if they are disciplined enough and try hard enough.

- It is your moral imperative to attain the ideal body and health at all costs, even at the expense of each other. And if that seems contradictory or impossible to you, well, that's probably a sign that you're not trying hard enough and are looking for excuses.

- If you struggle in your pursuit of pure wellness more than someone else, it can't be because their circumstances are different from yours. It's totally because you're a lazy piece of garbage. Stop making excuses. (And if someone else struggles more than you, then they are clearly not working as hard and not as good as you are. You should probably shame them.)

- If you're tired, that's good because you should work until you're tired! But it's also bad, because that means you're lazy and not fit enough.

- Oh, and your body's probably gross and you should be ashamed of it.

And then we're sent to gym class.

I don't know anyone who has come out of the North American physical education system unscathed. For most of us, gym was a place where teachers who may or may not have had a background in athletics, fitness, kinesiology, or health—or any interest in them—introduced us to a few sports-related skills and then threw us into endless competition. It sapped the life out of whatever enjoyment we were getting from moving our bodies as kids and injected a ton of steroids right into the ass of our teenage insecurities. Few if any of the hours we spent flinging balls at or around each other were dedicated to learning how our bodies worked and why, let alone how we might do things with our bodies that actually made us feel good.

Kids who excelled at gym learned that physical skills and fitness were inherent qualities that required no further understanding, maintenance, or care. Their self-esteem suffered as they grew older and started to experience physical challenges beyond their understanding and specific skill set. Those of us who sucked at PE fared even worse. We learned that physical skills and fitness were inherent qualities we were never going to have, and any attempt to attain them would result in deserved humiliation and scrutiny.

(One day in ninth grade, my extremely Over It teacher gave up, took us to the weight room, threw on a *Sweatin' to the Oldies* tape, and left us to our own devices. We were snarky mid-1990s teenagers, so we approached the exercise with our usual irony, but we ended up getting really into it. We danced. We giggled. A girl who had attacked me during our basketball unit because she didn't like my face smiled at me. I later realized that it was the first time we hadn't been pitted against each other or ourselves in gym class since kindergarten. And we'd flourished. Sometimes I wonder what would have happened if we'd been given that opportunity more often.)

For some people, such early experiences are enough to permanently destroy any interest they might have had in moving their bodies. Quite understandably, they tap out as soon as they complete their mandatory phys ed classes. Those who keep going or work up the nerve to try again have to deal with fitness culture in general, and the fitness industry in particular, which salts all of the wounds from our formative years. Or more accurately, it rips them open, pours an entire jar inside, and then shames us for our sodium consumption.

There are great people in fitness. There are great exercises that can help you achieve fantastic things. There are services and products that I find very useful, too. In fact, the fitness world has noticeably improved in my lifetime, largely thanks to the incredible work of marginalized trainers and influencers who have encouraged the industry to become less rigid and more inclusive. But there are also a lot of not-so-great people, exercises, and products. And even the good ones exist in the same world that has taught us all of those damaging opinions about health and wellness and went through the same early physical education that fractured our relationship with our bodies and their movements.

You will probably learn more about how your body works and why from the average training session or exercise resource than you did in the entirety of phys ed. But that's more an indictment of gym class than praise of gym culture. There is still a chance that you'll still be encouraged to push that body beyond its limits and hate it for some reason or other. Opportunities to treat our bodies well and to work with them instead of against them, or to treat them as something other than an enemy or a disobedient child, are still far and few between.

Every terrible lesson we've ever been taught about work, rest, food, and health is pushed to its extreme in gym culture. We're given increasingly narrow ideas of what a perfect body is and an endlessly shifting series of so-called perfect workouts that are supposed to help us achieve it. Anything less than perfect is considered a personal failing. Competition and judgment flourish. All our past insecurities are heightened by this onslaught of bad ideas and worse vibes, and then exploited by companies and individuals who want to sell us memberships and products. And the majority of what they're trying to sell us has been designed and implemented by people who were good at gym class. Most of whom are still working through their own issues, and don't have the best grasp of what physical education was like for the rest of us.

It's easy to get caught up in the fitness industry's unrelenting fixation with finding the best possible exercises, diets, and bodies. It's easier still to be confused by the constantly shifting goalposts of what constitutes "the best" within that world. Cardio is in one year and out the next. The ideal glute size keeps shifting. Even the perfect tightness for the pelvic floor has been in flux. These trends are especially counterproductive for anxious and depressed exercisers. Anxiety might cause you to freeze in the face of too much conflicting information and too many options. Depression might tell you to just give up, because what's the point of trying at all if it isn't going to be good enough anyway?

The fitness industry also has this ugly habit of taking perfectly good facts, blowing them out of proportion, selling people a bunch of shit based on these trumped-up promises, and then blaming individuals when they fail and leaving them with the fallout. Then the industry can double down on its outsize promises and capitalize on your feelings of failure to sell you more new shit.

For example, look at what they've done to the (accurate) claim we started with: "Exercise can help to reduce anxiety and depression symptoms." That's a very good thing! If you've ever struggled with anxiety, depression, or just feeling crummy, a potentially enjoyable practice that has a good shot at making you feel less awful is damn near a miracle. But somehow "help to reduce" keeps getting distorted into "cure," and far too many people in the fitness industry keep running with it, offering hot new workouts and gear that are supposed to fix everything that ails you. So now depressed and anxious people are stuck with people who have no business discussing their medical history telling them to ditch meds and therapy for dumbbells—not to mention busybodies barking "Have you tried yoga?" all the time.

(This is the only time I will mention medication in this book. It's not my area of expertise and it's also none of my business. Don't trust any fitness professional or training buddy who tries to tell you what you should or shouldn't be taking.)

And if you don't manage to squat the pain away, it couldn't possibly be because exercise isn't a one-size-fits-all solution to complicated personal and societal problems! It must be because you didn't work hard enough or well enough! Or because you were doing the wrong workout and didn't work hard enough to find the right one. Whatever the case, it's probably all your fault and you probably need to try harder and try this new perfect workout. It's so weird that you don't feel better yet, you lazy, pathetic piece of garbage!

There is no trainer you can hire, no class you can take, no workout you can try, no resource you can access, no role model you can look up to, and no support system you can reach out to that is wholly untouched by this mess. A lot of people at every level are doing their best to unlearn the harmful lessons they've been taught about health and build more constructive programs and

BUST THIS MYTH:
"NO EXCUSES"

You may have heard that there are no acceptable excuses for not engaging in hard exercise (and the related belief that there are no acceptable excuses for not engaging in self-punishment if you don't exercise hard). In fact, the opposite is true: anything is an acceptable excuse. There is no minimum amount of suffering required for you to deserve to be gentler with yourself. There's no magical line separating people whose difficulties getting into exercise stem from "real" issues from those having problems because they're lazy or bad. A lot of popular approaches to physical movement frustrate and alienate a lot of people for a lot of reasons. And they're all valid. You do not need to be THIS mentally ill to struggle with getting on this ride.

I have depression and anxiety and talk a lot about those issues, but you don't need a diagnosis to benefit from this idea. Any work you do as a result of the tips in this book isn't going to be negated if you're "only" sad, worried, or feeling off. And what's the worst that's going to happen if you take a day off from exercise because you feel moderately bad but not completely incapacitated? You get some rest, which everyone needs—we have a whole chapter on it starting on page 175—and you reinforce the idea that exercise can be something other than a slog and a punishment. Both of those have the potential to help your brain.

more inclusive spaces in fitness. But it does take effort to find those people and their work—and to determine which ones are going to be best for you and your needs. That effort can add another layer of stress to an already fraught situation.

Some people can thrive in these conditions. Others might succeed in spite of them, which is great for those people. Finding something in fitness that truly works for you isn't impossible. I don't want to take anything away from anyone who has managed it and I don't want to discourage anyone who is still trying. But I also don't want anyone who is struggling to blame themselves for what they're going through. A situation doesn't have to be completely insurmountable for it to completely suck.

IT FEELS HARD BECAUSE IT IS HARD

If you are struggling to find, start, and maintain regular physical activity to improve your life and mood, that's probably because the whole process can be very difficult, frustrating, and demoralizing. Plus, it might inadvertently reinforce a buttload of wretched things that depression, anxiety, and our dysfunctional society have been telling you about yourself.

It's hard to carry the weight of all your past experiences every time you try to take a step. It's hard to push back against the lifetime of destructive messages floating around in your head. And it's hard to find exercises, guidance, and communities that will actually help you in your efforts and not end up making things worse. Doing all of this would be a challenge if you were in perfect mental health, if such a thing exists. It becomes far more difficult when you're not.

These aren't excuses. They're 100 percent legitimate explanations.

Maybe it's a bit overwhelming to see the extent of the odds against you laid out so plainly, but I hope it's validating, too. I know all too well how depression and anxiety can make you doubt and blame yourself—and how many people who don't have to live your life will shamelessly doubt and blame you, too. Sometimes you might feel like you need an outside perspective to confirm that what you're going through isn't all in your head, to give you permission to believe yourself (or to tell those other people to shut up).

So here is my expert opinion as someone with a strong professional background in fitness and an even more extensive background in working out while depressed and anxious as hell. Use as necessary. Return to it as many times as you need to. Shove it in the face of anyone who gives you a hard time if that helps:

YOUR ISSUES WITH EXERCISE ARE REAL.
YOU'RE NOT WEAK OR PATHETIC.
YOU'RE NOT OVERREACTING.
YOU'RE NOT THE WORST.
YOU'RE NOT UNIQUELY BAD AT SOMETHING THAT COMES
EASILY TO EVERYONE ELSE ON THE PLANET.
YOU ARE DEFINITELY NOT ALONE.

And you're not stuck, either. Moving your body—or working up the nerve to try moving your body—does not always have to be this hard. You won't feel the way you're feeling right now forever. You can chip away at all of those lies, you can begin to heal the wounds they've left you with, and you can build something new in their place that will actually be good for you.

You have my permission—and my encouragement—to ignore any tip, suggestion, or idea related to fitness that stands in the way of you achieving that. Your goal is to feel better than you do right now. Anything that negates any improvements you're making or makes you feel worse is officially a contraindicated exercise.

Screw any attempts to moralize health and fitness. There's nothing inherently good about being in shape, whatever that means. If there were an inarguable standard of ideal wellness, you still wouldn't owe it to anyone to try to achieve it. But it doesn't exist, so you don't have to worry about that. You sure as hell don't owe anyone any effort to contort yourself into their perception of what wellness means, or what you should look or feel like, or what you should do with your time.

THE ONLY THING THAT MATTERS IS HOW YOU FEEL

Maybe the most important (and probably one of the hardest) steps is to give up on the idea of perfection. The perfect exercise is one that you will actually entertain the thought of doing. The perfect body is a breathing one. Anything that serves those ends is worth considering. Everything else is noise. Keep the information and the messages that work for you and chuck the rest. That includes the advice in this book—up to and including the advice that exercise can help you feel better. Seriously. You don't *have* to exercise. You can just read this book for the jokes.

Every time you start planning a new workout or new training regimen, think about why you want to try it. If you're doing it for your health, that's great. If it's something you used to like doing and you think you might enjoy doing it again if you can just push through the misery and inertia? That works, too. But if you're just doing it because you think you *should*, or if it becomes just another way to punish yourself, that doesn't work. If you can't come up with a single plan where the risk inherent in the attempt itself won't outweigh any benefit you might get from it, then don't do it. Take a break from the very idea of exercise and come back to it again in a few days to see if your perspective has changed. Exercise can't help with your anxiety or depression if even thinking about exercise makes you more anxious and depressed.

You'll probably need to spend the rest of your life essentially deprogramming yourself, because that's how pervasive and powerful our society's trash takes on wellness are. But every time you realize that someone or something is full of crap, and every time you remember that you don't have to put up with it, that lifelong effort gets a little easier. Hopefully it can make you be a little easier on yourself, too.

Developing a filter that will enable you to reject bad health-related information and keep the good—and minimize the harm that the bad information can cause you—is a lot like developing muscle or cardiovascular capacity. It takes a lot of repetition to build it and maintain it. But each time you put in that effort, you get a bit stronger. To help you get there, this book includes suggestions for how to change your perspective right alongside more common training tips.

If you're feeling overwhelmed or discouraged right now, here's something else to keep in mind: nothing you've read in this chapter is new. Maybe it's the first time that you've seen all the obstacles to finding, starting, and maintaining the right physical activity for you and your mental health laid out this way. Or the first time someone has confirmed that this is all real and you're not too sensitive, lazy, or making things up. But everything I've just broken down? You are already living it. And, despite all of it, something made you pick up this book and want to try.

You are already doing a good job.

THE RIGHT EXERCISE FOR YOU

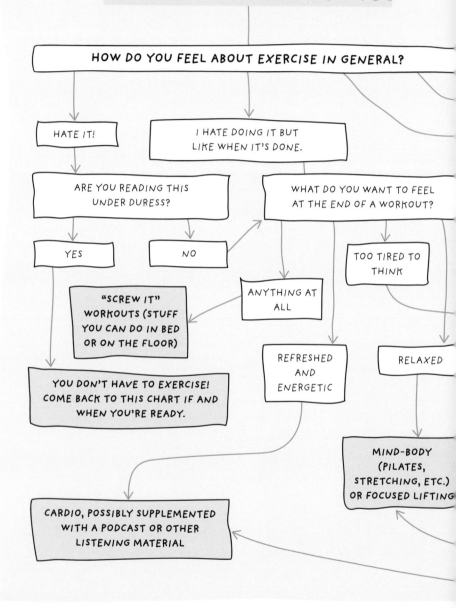

HOW DO YOU FEEL ABOUT EXERCISE IN GENERAL?

HATE IT!

I HATE DOING IT BUT LIKE WHEN IT'S DONE.

ARE YOU READING THIS UNDER DURESS?

WHAT DO YOU WANT TO FEEL AT THE END OF A WORKOUT?

YES

NO

TOO TIRED TO THINK

"SCREW IT" WORKOUTS (STUFF YOU CAN DO IN BED OR ON THE FLOOR)

ANYTHING AT ALL

YOU DON'T HAVE TO EXERCISE! COME BACK TO THIS CHART IF AND WHEN YOU'RE READY.

REFRESHED AND ENERGETIC

RELAXED

MIND-BODY (PILATES, STRETCHING, ETC.) OR FOCUSED LIFTING

CARDIO, POSSIBLY SUPPLEMENTED WITH A PODCAST OR OTHER LISTENING MATERIAL

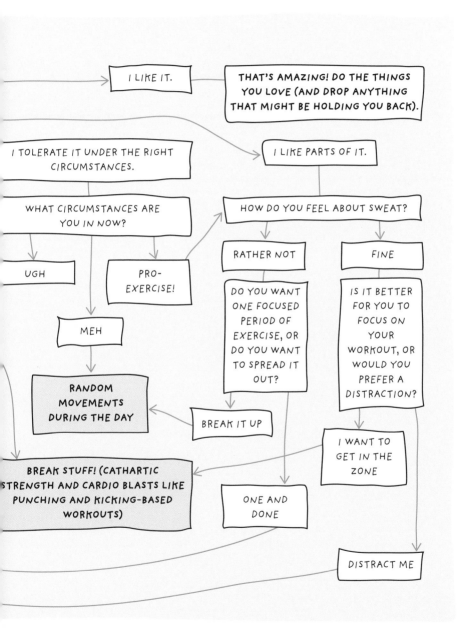

I LIKE IT.

THAT'S AMAZING! DO THE THINGS YOU LOVE (AND DROP ANYTHING THAT MIGHT BE HOLDING YOU BACK).

I TOLERATE IT UNDER THE RIGHT CIRCUMSTANCES.

I LIKE PARTS OF IT.

WHAT CIRCUMSTANCES ARE YOU IN NOW?

HOW DO YOU FEEL ABOUT SWEAT?

RATHER NOT

FINE

UGH

PRO-EXERCISE!

DO YOU WANT ONE FOCUSED PERIOD OF EXERCISE, OR DO YOU WANT TO SPREAD IT OUT?

IS IT BETTER FOR YOU TO FOCUS ON YOUR WORKOUT, OR WOULD YOU PREFER A DISTRACTION?

MEH

RANDOM MOVEMENTS DURING THE DAY

BREAK IT UP

BREAK STUFF! (CATHARTIC STRENGTH AND CARDIO BLASTS LIKE PUNCHING AND KICKING-BASED WORKOUTS)

I WANT TO GET IN THE ZONE

ONE AND DONE

DISTRACT ME

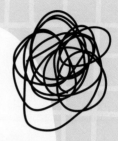

– TWO –

GET MOVING—
OR AT LEAST
GET UP

How to get started when you'd
rather lie down

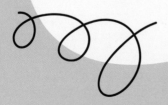

When I was taking my first personal-instructor training course in the mid-2000s, I was taught that most of my clients would come to us because they reached a breaking point. That they would only choose to exercise when the discomfort of not moving their bodies outweighed anything we might put them through. Fifteen years of life and work experience later, I have yet to see any evidence of this point. Frankly, I think framing the barrier between inaction and action this way, and, especially, developing training techniques based on this theory, is at best ill-informed and yet more evidence that most fitness programs are designed and run by people who excelled in gym class. At worst, I think it's condescending drivel that borders on victim blaming. *Oh, you still haven't started exercising? Maybe you aren't suffering enough yet!*

I won't discount the possibility that someone might hit rock-bottom, decide exercise is the lesser of two evils, experience an epiphany, and live and move happily ever after. But this has never happened to me, or any of the people I've worked with. There are times when being in my own head is worse than doing a hundred burpees, and that is still not, in and of itself, enough to get me out of bed.

So I'd like to propose an alternate theory: getting started is just plain hard. It doesn't matter how bad you feel before you get going, or how good you know you'll feel after. It doesn't matter what is on either side of the starting line. Crossing it is still a Herculean task.

This is true about starting things in general, not just exercise. It can be something allegedly small like getting out of bed and starting your day, or big like launching a new project or setting a major life change in motion. You still have to wrap your head around what you're about to do, manage whatever complicated mix of procrastination/fear of failure/anxiety about new things/ lack of energy/lack of fucks you've got going on, and overcome inertia in order to take those first steps.

The average exercise regimen is full of stuff that needs starting. You have to start doing physical activity in a general sense. But once you've managed that, you still have to start each individual workout. Depending on the type of exercise you pick, you might also have to begin multiple sets of movements within a single workout. In better times, this whole process can be a touch draining. When you're depressed, it can feel insurmountable. No amount of Nike sloganeering is going to make it any easier to just do.

Based on that theory, here is a list of actions I recommend taking right from the top:

- Give yourself credit for every time you have successfully started something. Get as small and specific as you need to give yourself whatever validation you need and remind yourself that you are capable of getting things done. You woke up today. That's important. You decided to read this and you're doing that right now. Amazing!

- Give yourself a break for the times you've struggled to start. This is hard.

- Give yourself a break for anything you managed to launch with relative ease before that feels far less possible now. We've already established that this is hard. When you managed it before, you were doing something great. But that doesn't mean it's easy, and there are any number of normal reasons why your capacity might fluctuate. Maybe the task you're trying to start isn't the right one for you right now. Or maybe you need a different approach or a little outside help. Whatever the problem is, it's not something fundamental about you.

- Break the task(s) you are trying to start into smaller pieces. As small as you need to make them until they start to feel manageable.

- Eliminate or minimize any barriers to attempting these small chunks that you're able to.

- Try.

- If you succeed, give yourself credit.

- If you're still struggling, give yourself a break. Sure, some people require a tough-love approach, but if you found it motivating to talk shit about yourself, you'd probably have finished your workout (and your novel, and your meal prep) by now. Why not try a gentler approach?

- Regroup and reframe the tasks as necessary. Is there something about the size or type of the tasks that's not doing it for you? Is there something about the way you're thinking about the tasks that is making them more difficult for you to face? Take a pause, don't beat yourself up for needing that pause, and then think about what changes might help you cross your starting line.

- Try again when you're ready.

I'll dig into how you can break up individual exercises and ways to piece them together into modular workouts in Chapter 4, "Break It Up." But first, I'm going to focus on how you can approach everything from the first step to the last set, starting with the big picture and working down to the most practical everyday concerns. Not all of this information is going to be useful for everyone. Depending on your circumstances and the way you're wired, some of it might end up being the exact opposite. So I'm also going to provide a heads-up for what parts you might want to skip, why they might not be the best for you, and where you can pick up again.

First I'll look at how to get into—or back into—exercise in the most general sense. I'll be going over different ways to get started, what types of people they're most suitable for, and what you can do if absolutely nothing I suggest sounds remotely appealing or possible. It's unlikely that I will be telling you anything groundbreaking in this section. Again, exercise isn't new. You know what a gym is. But I've found it helpful to take this kind of overview when I'm planning my own training. Doing so allows me to clarify what I'm looking for and where I'm most likely to find it, and it's a great mental exercise for reinforcing that fitness is something that needs to suit me, not the other way around.

Then I'll tackle how you can get into each individual workout, and what to do if none of those tips are enough for you.

GETTING STARTED: THE BIG PICTURE

If you find motivation in making plans, or if you prefer to prepare for a new undertaking by working through every possible option and scenario, the next few pages will break down some possibilities for creating a new, improved approach to exercise. If you're in a headspace where things like making longer-term plans or conceiving of a future at all are more likely to overwhelm you and make you freeze than encourage you in any way, you can skip it and proceed to page 49, where we'll talk about winging it.

In the broadest terms, there are two ways you can get into exercise that involve any kind of structure or plan: either you pay for a new service or product (or a combination of the two), or you piece together a routine based on resources already at your disposal. The first option includes gym memberships, classes, personal training sessions, at-home workout equipment, and equipment that comes with a built-in instruction component (Peloton, Mirror, etc.). The second can include any combination of condo or community gyms, outdoor spaces, a spare corner of your house or your bed, workout videos on YouTube or other streaming services, workout buddies, random equipment you might own from past flirtations with exercise, household items you've MacGuyvered into exercise equipment (the first weights I ever lifted were soup cans), and your own body.

There are advantages and disadvantages to both approaches. I'm going to cover the basic pros and cons to help you figure out which one is most in line with your goals and needs.

MAKING AN INVESTMENT

If price isn't an issue for you, or if needing to get the full value out of something once you've paid for it is a useful source of motivation, this avenue could have potential. If you can't afford to pay for memberships, training, or gear, or if worrying about making the right investments and getting enough value from your workouts runs the risk of outweighing any anti-anxiety benefits you'll get from them, then you can move on to other options. There are plenty of low-budget and free alternatives that can be just as good for your brain and body while being much better for your budget and peace of mind. (If money issues bother you and make you feel like giving up or shutting down, I strongly encourage you to head straight to "DIY," on page 42—you've learned everything you need to know!)

There is also an emotional and mental cost to consider when you're taking this path. There are tons of great gyms, trainers, and products out there, but finding them can be a crapshoot. All the problems with the fitness industry that we talked about in the Chapter 1 still exist, and it will probably take effort to navigate the harmful stuff and find what's right for you—or to develop the ability to tune it out and do your own thing in a suboptimal environment. If you have the bandwidth to do this kind of research and prep upfront, though, it is possible to find the right venue and people for you—and once you do, you'll be able to redirect the energy you put toward research into getting the most out of your new investment.

Personal trainers and group fitness instructors can also tell you what to do and when to do it, a role that personal training services love to brand as hardline accountability. You're paying someone to tell you what to do, and that makes you responsible to them and your wallet. This concept clearly works for a lot of people, because it's been a popular selling point for decades. But I worry that this perspective alienates as many people as it attracts. What about those who already feel like they're crumbling under the weight of their responsibilities? If you're in that category, I recommend looking at the situation the way one of my favorite clients laid it out when she first hired me.

One day, she started taking a methodical account of everything she needed and wanted to do in her daily life, including work, chores, hobbies, socializing, etc. Then she thought about how much time and energy she realistically had to tackle them. From there, she sorted things into tasks she could handle on her own and tasks that might require outside assistance. For her, exercise was something that had a meaningful impact on her physical and mental well-being, but did not inspire her in any way whatsoever. She probably could have forced herself to research workouts, and put together her own routines, but hiring a personal trainer enabled her to spend that time and mental effort on other activities that were better suited to her energy level, skill set, and interests. She didn't need someone to answer to. She needed someone to assist her. It was basically the thought process that goes into hiring another person to change the oil in your car, even though you could almost certainly do it yourself if you watched enough YouTube tutorials.

Group fitness, dance, or martial arts classes and the general atmosphere of a moderately populated gym are also good sources of outside motivation if you're the kind of person who is enriched by socializing, community, and the feeling that you're in something together. (Or if you're someone who finds peer pressure to be a positive influence.) They are not the best choice for people who would prefer not to be perceived while exercising. Meanwhile, at-home personal training services and virtual instruction are solid alternatives for anyone who wants the guidance and encouragement of gym-based

BUST THIS MYTH:
"STAY POSITIVE"

My favorite workout videos ever are the Rushfit series by Georges St-Pierre. The exercises are great, but what keeps me coming back is watching this Ultimate Fighting Championship legend grimace through the workouts and laugh about how little he's enjoying himself. I find it extremely encouraging. If one of the fittest men on the planet is struggling with a move, then it's OK for me to struggle and bitch about it, too.

Good attitudes and eternally perky instructors clearly work for some people, or they wouldn't be so damned unavoidable. But a so-called good attitude isn't for everyone and is not a prerequisite for getting going or getting stuff done. It's wonderful if you have positive reasons to move your body and feel positive things while you're doing it, but it's just as fine if you feel the opposite. Train out of spite or insolence! Be amiably miserable about it like GSP! Stomp through it with a begrudging sense of purpose like the people who made all of those "going for a silly little walk for my silly little mental health" TikToks and Instagram reels during the pandemic lockdown!

Physical activity can be cathartic, so there's a good chance you'll end up taking the edge off whatever "bad" attitude or emotion motivated you to start. (But if it doesn't, it's OK to feel sad and angry about that, too.)

sessions and classes without all the people.

Personal training and group instruction work well for people who require some level of externally imposed structure. They require you to be at a certain place at a certain time. Commercial gyms are also a good option for structure, because you have to fit your workouts into work hours, unless you're lucky enough to have access to a twenty-four-hour location. Those parameters can be limiting and challenging—or just a plain bummer—for anyone who needs flexibility in their workout plans for any reason ranging from work and life demands to personal preference.

Investing in new workout equipment is a good option for people who are inspired by novelty. And your home can be a great place to start if you're feeling unsure of yourself or completely done with everyone else.

If you're so inclined, you can put together your own workout plans and train completely on your own. I'll be getting into that approach in more detail in Chapter 4, "Break It Up." If you're not interested in or ready for that level of self-direction, the growing world of virtual instruction offers you an excellent mix of gym and home training. You get all the professional expertise and most of the external guidance of being in a gym setting, but with a somewhat more flexible schedule and none of the other people.

The most obvious and accessible form of virtual training is the aforementioned subscription-based equipment. This one-stop-shopping option is useful for anyone who doesn't want to put much thought into their home gym setup. All you have to do is research which product will work best for you; when you choose, you get the instruction and the equipment all at once. Once you're set up, you can either pick one type of class and stick with it or explore all the options available in your own time and at your own pace. (If you're not the most assertive person on the planet, this is also a good way to test out exercises you might be curious about without trying to please an in-person instructor and potentially getting stuck doing things you don't want to do.)

For those who don't want to commit to bigger equipment or a subscription, prefer a more personal touch, or want to give their money to smaller businesses, you can also look into a less formal or corporate arrangement, like hiring a personal trainer to coach you through Zoom sessions.

If you live in a small space and are bothered by clutter, if you feel guilty when you buy things for yourself, or if the very idea of fitness equipment bores you to tears, though, the stress and the buzzkill you're likely to experience with this option would likely outweigh the good it would do you.

DIY

Of course, you don't need to invest in or commit to anything new to start exercising. There's a whole world of exercise opportunities that are either already available to you or easily accessible.

This route offers obvious financial benefits. It's an excellent alternative if you don't have the cash, find money a source of distress, or simply prefer to spend your disposable income on things you like more. But it is also a good plan of attack for anyone looking for a flexible and low-pressure entry into physical activity. That includes self-directed learners, introverts, night owls, and anyone who would prefer to stay as far away as possible from any hint of formalized fitness culture.

The biggest concern with going your own way is the mental effort involved. In order to plan and execute a DIY exercise routine, you will have to drum up your own initial interest, do your own research to figure out what you want to do and how you should do it, source your own facilities and gear, and muster your own motivation to follow through.

If you're a task-oriented person or if learning new things invigorates you, this method could end up working well. There can be unexpected benefits to forging your own way, too. When I first started exercising as an adult, I couldn't afford much more than a book on Pilates and a copy of Frederic Delavier's *Women's Strength Training Anatomy*. I was mostly interested in having more defined biceps and abs, but learning about my muscles and how I could make them bigger ended up having a positive influence on my relationship to my body. The more I understood about how it worked and why, the more I was able to appreciate it—and occasionally, when I was really lucky, be kinder to it.

If you're not into that kind of effort and the reward doesn't sound sufficient, though, you're not out of luck. There are plenty of resources online, in your community, and in your local library that can ease at least a portion of your sourcing and planning load. Using those resources, you'll be able to find everything from tips on how to find and make equipment to free, complete workout plans and videos, which will tell you exactly what to do and give you guidance about when and how to do it.

Depending on where you live, you might have access to free or low-fee training facilities. If you can't or don't want to join a commercial gym, but you like the idea of having a place to go to do stuff, I suggest looking into community alternatives. Do you live in an apartment or condo that has a gym space? If you're a student, does your school offer access to its sports facilities? Are there community centers nearby that have exercise equipment? Do you know anyone with a home gym setup they'd be willing to open up to you? (For the last one, make sure it's someone you're comfortable with and know well, since you'll be taking your first fledgling steps toward working out in their space—a vulnerable moment.)

Unless you happen to be buddies with a benevolent rich muscle nerd, none of the above choices are likely to have brand new, top-of-the-line equipment. But you don't need anything fancy to get a good and rewarding workout, especially not when you're getting started. And what these options might lack in gear, they often make up in atmosphere. I've worked out and taught in everything from the prissiest tennis clubs to places that could have been featured in *Rocky* training montages, and free or very-low-cost weight rooms have been the most low-pressure and judgment-free environments I've encountered. People in building gyms tend to leave one another alone. People in community gyms will usually leave you alone or give you some mix of guidance and encouragement, and will either come through with useful support or politely back off depending on whether or not you're interested in what they're offering. It's not impossible to find these vibes in pricier gyms, but more accessible spaces seem to offer it far more consistently. (School gyms have been hit or miss for me. But if your school has more than one facility, I recommend giving the smaller or older one a shot. They tend to be more relaxed and populated with like-minded people.)

If you don't have access to an established workout space, or if you don't want it, you have the great outdoors to consider. (Weather and climate permitting, of course. As someone with an allergy to cold temperatures who lives in Canada, I am painfully aware of the limitations of this choice.) This includes abundant resources like sidewalks, trails, or a patch of grass in a park. Some parks also have dedicated fitness trails and equipment like pull-up bars, parallel bars, obstacle courses, calisthenics courses, and outdoor weight and cardio machines. And some of those come complete with workout plans/suggestions posted at each station, which takes the whole planning part off your plate. (A quick search for fitness trails or outdoor gyms in your area should point you in the right direction.)

You can also get creative with other spaces in your general area. Cemeteries are excellent for walks, runs, and interval training. Other than remote trails, they're the quietest public place where you can exercise, and their paths are usually made of asphalt, which is kinder on joints than concrete sidewalks. Empty playground equipment can be used for strength training, cardio drills, and assisted stretching. As long as you treat the place and the other people in it with respect and common sense (e.g., quietly walk past funerals, avoid working out on jungle gyms when kids are playing on them), almost anything can be used for exercise.

Outdoor workouts are great for people who are motivated by having a specific place to go do something separate from whatever else they're doing, people whose preferred types of exercise require more space than they have at home, people who like being outside, and people who don't like being outside

YOUR FITNESS FIT

If you're feeling unmotivated, drained, or overwhelmed, the very idea of having to put on clothes in the morning may be too much to handle— let *alone* the perception that you need to have special clothes to exercise in. Fortunately, workout gear isn't as complicated as it may seem. Here's what matters, and what doesn't.

IMPORTANT

- Does not pull or chafe in a way that keeps you from moving well
- Provides adequate support for bouncy parts
- Won't cause you to be so overheated or so chilled that it makes activity harder
- Has pocket(s) if you need to keep your keys, phone, etc., on you while exercising
- Makes you feel cool (not essential, but a nice bonus)

NOT IMPORTANT

- Brand name
- Matching set
- Technology like "moisture wicking" fabric (nice but not necessary!)
- Looks like exercise clothes
- Makes other people think you look cool

but tolerate it. Fresh air and sunlight and all that crap are, I begrudgingly admit, at least 20 percent to 50 percent as refreshing, head-clearing, and spirit-lifting as overbearing nature lovers make it sound. Taking it outside isn't the best choice if you can't or don't want to leave your house, if having to go to a second location to do something feels like an insurmountable hurdle, or if there's still too much risk of being perceived out there.

That brings us home—which happens to be my personal favorite training venue. Of course, the average residence has limitations as a training facility. Unless you happen to have a state-of-the-art home gym lying around, you probably won't be hitting a lot of lifting, distance, or speed-based personal bests there. If I woke up tomorrow and decided that I wanted to pursue body-building, I'd have to join a gym again. If I didn't have the knowledge base I have now and wasn't comfortable getting all my information from videos, books, and websites, I would need to venture outside occasionally to procure some in-person feedback. And if I had a greater need for social interaction than I do, I'd probably need to leave my house to source some in-person *anything*.

I'm also mindful of the fact that not everyone lives somewhere that is good for their mental health, let alone somewhere where they can launch a campaign to improve it. I can't imagine that I'd be able to do much for my physical or mental health in a place where I didn't feel physically or mentally safe. If my home workouts were regularly interrupted by more than the occasional visit from my cat, I would need to go elsewhere to carve out some time and space for myself.

But as someone who has exercised at home both out of necessity and choice—and who specialized in clients who preferred to work out in their own homes—I'm familiar with its underrated potential, too.

The biggest benefit of staying home is that it grants you an incredible amount of freedom to go at your own pace. This goes for everything from learning how to do an individual move to piecing together ways to conceive of physical movement as something other than a source of pain and shame.

I apologize if the following anecdote is sappy, but it is about something that changed my life in a way even I can't be cynical about. I started lifting those soup cans I mentioned in my late teens because I couldn't afford a gym membership, but even if I could have I think I would have been too terrified to actually go. As a kid I was uncoordinated and I got something I called "gym breath" when our teachers sent us outside to run (I later learned that the medical term for gym breath is exercise-induced asthma), and my fondest memories of phys ed were the times I had a sick note. I was ashamed of what I considered my past exercise failures, and extremely intimidated by anyone I perceived to be more successful.

My childhood bedroom ended up becoming a kind of incubator for my tiny, fledgling interest in fitness. I got to work with few time constraints, very little pressure, and no audience. There was no one around to judge or pity me, and no one to whom I could neurotically compare myself and my progress. I think my makeshift weights ended up tricking my brain into relaxing a bit, too; it wasn't perfect equipment, so I didn't have to be perfect, either. That was exactly the environment I needed to begin figuring my shit out. Many of my at-home clients had their own unpleasant experiences that made them just as hesitant to begin formalized fitness as I'd been, if not more so. Being able to carve out their own space separate from anything that had hurt or alienated them made a world of difference to them, too.

If you're not into the touchy-feely side of home exercise, it has plenty of practical benefits, too. You don't have to commute anywhere, which saves time and eliminates a potential barrier to getting started. You don't have to work up the nerve to leave your house, travel somewhere, arrive at your location, *and then* work out. You go straight to the workout. You don't even have to get dressed if you don't want to.

If you find being around a lot of other people anxiety inducing or draining, staying home can spare you the energy you'd spend on traveling to, from, and through another workout destination and navigating crowds along the way. If you have sensory issues, you might find it easier to manage your needs in a smaller and quieter space that you have more control over.

This option is also great for people seeking flexibility in their fitness routines. From the comfort of your home, you can do your workout at any time and in almost any configuration. You can schedule it for off hours if that's better for your body's natural rhythms. You can fly by the seat of your pants and throw in a workout when you find a spare moment and a crumb of motivation. Or you can do little bits of it over the course of the day. You can roll out of bed and do something. You can even stay in bed and try some stuff. You don't have to get dressed for that, either.

For obvious reasons, I would not recommend this mildly feral stay-at-home fitness lifestyle if you function better under externally imposed deadlines, pressure, or encouragement. If you do need outside accountability but you're committed to the home-based lifestyle, I'd suggest finding someone you can check in with and answer to as needed. But if the outside world is more likely to be a source of stress, demoralization, or plain annoyance than a source of support, you might be pleasantly surprised by how much better you can feel when you shut it out for a few reps. Even if you don't love the reps themselves.

MIXING AND MATCHING

I haven't covered every single pro and con of the above workout possibilities, but this should be enough to give you an idea of what options are out there. There's no perfect choice, but there's no wrong choice either. It's all about what might work for you, your body, and your circumstances.

If one of the scenarios that you've read above—or something entirely different that you've come up with on your own—genuinely appeals to you, I recommend capitalizing on that enthusiasm and going for it. If one or more options seem OK-ish, you could make use of free trial options that many gyms and workout plans offer and test them out. If that's too much, you can always keep those options in the back of your mind, start with something more accessible, and give them a try if and when you're ready. If nothing really appeals to you, but you found something you wouldn't hate, that's worth a shot.

None of the choices you're making have to be permanent. If you start something and it doesn't work out, you don't have to do it forever. You can quit. You can try other things. You can take a break and regroup if you need to. This doesn't mean that you've failed or that you're starting from square one. Your goal is to try to feel better and something about it wasn't doing that for you. It failed you, not the other way around. And you're not starting over, either. You took those daunting first steps, and whatever you do next will be another step that builds on what you've already experienced and learned. Even if that lesson is "Ugh, I'm never doing *that* again." Discovering what demotivates you can be a part of figuring out what motivates you.

I know that this is all much easier for me to say than for you to take to heart. There are still times when I struggle to apply this advice to myself. But I promise you it's the truth. It's not even sugarcoated. This is a totally practical and functional approach to the goals you're pursuing.

WINGING IT

Of course, you don't need to make a plan before you start. You also don't need to set long-term goals, or even short-term ones beyond "I think I'm going to do a thing." Hell, it's not 100 percent necessary that you have any clue what kind of movement you're going to do until a few minutes before you do it.

All you need in order to wing it is a little bit of willingness to do something and a thing to do. If you find that you have some time, energy and desire, pick a thing and go for it.

The thing can be small, like taking a walk around the block and seeing where that goes. Or it can be bigger, like thinking that you've always been curious about boxing, impulse-googling gyms near you, signing up for a trial class, and going. It can be of almost any duration and intensity. The dimensions of the Band-Aid don't matter nearly as much as the fact that you're pulling it off.

(I can't stop you from jumping straight into an advanced workout, but I am going to strongly caution against it if you've been inactive for any period of time. The best-case scenario is that you spend the next couple of days sore and possibly discouraged. The worst case is that you hurt yourself. In addition to the obvious harm this will do to your health, it can also put a real damper on your enthusiasm to try again. Hard workouts that you might have done before can still pose a risk to your current well-being. Speaking from experience, it's far more beneficial—and less humbling—to slowly build back to your previous activity level than it is to jump right back in, fail to magically pick up where you left off, and wallow in almost inevitable self-flagellation.)

You might be surprised at where a single impromptu workout can take you. My mom's running career began with a walk. After a lifetime of cycling through workout plans that failed her, she decided she wanted something different, fished a pair of old shoes out of the basement, and took them outside. When that went OK, she took them for another lap the next day. And the next. Once she'd established a routine, she started adding distance and experimenting with pace. Out of curiosity, she started running a few steps at a time. She liked that, so she added more. At that point, she started to research running and responsibly built her way to up to running 5 kilometers (3.1 miles). Then 10 kilometers (6.2 miles). Then she started doing half and full marathons for fun. All because she woke up one day and felt like doing something.

But that first step doesn't need to lead to life-changing transformation in order to help you feel better. It can also lead to a perfectly good regular-ish routine. (I'd still be proudly sharing my mom's example as a success story if "all" she'd done was continue to wake up and choose to walk.) It can also lead to a loosely connected series of impromptu undertakings—which isn't far from what was keeping me afloat as I wrote this book. I randomly chose what

I'd like to do on good days. I figured out what I was most willing and able to do on the not so good ones, including rest. Most of the time, I did it. But if I didn't? Bonus rest day.

Wherever winging it takes you, the important thing is that you started something and you did it. Or at least part of it. You got the obvious benefits of the physical activity you were doing, and you might have received some perspective out of the deal. If anxiety was telling you that doing the thing was worse than anticipating it, your anxiety was wrong. If depression was telling you that your efforts would never lead to results, it was wrong. And if they were wrong about those simple facts, maybe they were wrong about other things, too.

GETTING STARTED: THE DAY-TO-DAY

Unfortunately, not everything is going to be smooth sailing after you take those first steps. That doesn't mean that every single workout is going to be an insurmountable struggle—once you've made that massive effort to start, subsequent workouts will most likely start to seem more approachable and manageable. And the more movement you do, the more proof you have that you *can* do it. But even the perkiest and most determined fitness buff has off days. It's perfectly normal to feel unmotivated, tired, or bored sometimes. And it's probably going to happen more frequently if you're already existing in a constant state of panic, feeling like a hollow shell of yourself, or both.

When I'm feeling too overwhelmed or exhausted to exercise, or I simply don't want to, I find that it helps to break up every part of my workout—including scheduling, preparation, and cleanup—into the smallest pieces possible. If after doing that the pieces are still giving me trouble, I also look at different ways I can approach them and different ways I can encourage myself to try them.

Here are some examples:

Work with your natural schedule (and don't feel guilty about it). When planning a workout, you will most likely need to keep in mind your other commitments and the time constraints of whatever resources you're using. What you don't have to consider, though, is any notion of when is the "right" time to exercise, or any of the weird ways our society moralizes early birds and romanticizes getting up at four a.m. to cram in a five a.m. cycling class before work. (It's great if that works for you, but there's nothing wrong with you if it doesn't!)

Figuring out when you actually have time to exercise is important, but so is figuring out when you have the energy to do it. If your answer is different from fitness norms, so be it. Work out at odd hours. Break your workout into even smaller pieces and do little bits of it scattered throughout the day. If you randomly stumble across an extra bit of drive during your off hours, throw in some extra movement you enjoy. It can be a structured exercise like push-ups if you're into that, but it can also be a one-person dance party.

If you're worried that taking this approach means that you're babying yourself or not taking exercise seriously enough, remember that learning to adapt to and work with your body's natural rhythms is something that professional athletes do all the time. For an extreme example, there's a professional wrestler named Tetsuya Naito who regularly works out at three a.m. He's a natural night owl and feels too wired to sleep after nighttime events, anyway, so he takes care of his weights and cardio in the middle of the night.

Everything I've said about respecting your body's schedule and rhythm also applies to the pace at which you do your workouts and the progress you see from them. Do what works for you and don't worry about the rest. (I know this is easier said than done. But if it helps to have a person with fitness expertise give you permission, you just got it.)

Remove as many potential obstacles as you can. Exercise can be daunting enough when you're not feeling your best. When you add preparation and cleanup to the mix, it can quickly start to feel like way too much to even bother trying. When I'm in that state, I find it helpful to reconsider how much I *really* need to do before and after my workout, and when I *really* need to do it.

If the act of getting changed into workout gear feels like too much effort, think about workarounds that are comfortable for you. Can you wear a sports bra to work and head straight to a cardio session after? What about sleeping in some of your gear, rolling out of bed, and waking up with some stretching? If that still feels like a pain in the ass, what about working out in what you're already wearing? Casual clothes and office wear aren't the most comfortable thing you'll ever move in, but I wouldn't say it's any less pleasant than climbing through mud as part of an obstacle course race, and that's a socially accepted thing that people do all the time in the name of being fit and tough. There was a regular at my old gym who always trained in a white dress shirt and khakis. Did people notice? Sure. I did a double take at first. Did some people comment on it? Probably. But after a while, all most of us noticed was that he was always there and he seemed pretty damned content to be doing his business-casual cardio.

If the idea of showering immediately after exercising feels like too much work on top of everything else, or if you know you won't have the energy to work out *and* shower, can you temporarily put showering out of your mind? Sometimes I promise myself that I can consider my hygiene options after I'm finished. I usually do feel like a shower when I'm done, because I don't enjoy the sensation of being sweaty, and I find the water soothing after hard training. Depending on what kind of exercise you're doing, it might be a necessity. (If you're participating in contact combat sports, for example, showering is an important part of preventing ringworm and staph.) But if you're not in one of those categories, you might be able to have a little more flexibility in your routine.

If setting up for a home workout is a brain block for you, do you have the space to leave a piece of equipment ready to go? I currently have a suspension trainer hanging in my hallway. Setting it up is hardly a laborious process—it takes about thirty seconds to do safely—but I'm going through a real out of sight, out of mind phase. If I don't see it right in front of me, I'm not going to think about it, let alone dig it out and use it. When it's in my face, I find myself thinking about the kind of stuff I'd like to do with it—and then doing it. Sometimes I stop to do a few sets when the mood hits me.

Just take a bite. If a whole workout is too intimidating, start with a warm-up and see how much you can add to it after that. There's a good chance you'll feel like continuing once you're already moving. But if you don't, you've still completed a decent warm-up.

Bribe yourself. When nothing else is getting you going, I see nothing wrong with a little bit of a material reward. If it's in your budget, you can promise yourself that you'll buy something you've really wanted when you finish an especially hard workout. But small treats work, too. Sometimes I use stickers because that childhood reward rush still works for me. (While you can use almost anything to bribe yourself to exercise, I would strongly caution against using food. Fitness is already so weird and so toxic about diet, and treating sustenance as a special treat you get for getting your reps in could hurt you more than it might help.)

Have backup plans. Don't be afraid to use them. I have lifelong issues with all-or-nothing thinking, so I'm painfully aware of how easy it is to assume that everything's ruined if you can't do the workout you had scheduled or mapped out in your head. But I also know from experience that it is *not* actually the end of the world, no matter how much it feels like it at the time. There's absolutely nothing wrong with saying "screw it" and taking another rest day. If you'd prefer to have other options you can fall back on, though, it helps to keep have a few go-to alternate plans. If you can't face the gym, what about going for a walk? If you can't bear to leave the house, what about putting on a workout video and seeing how that feels? If you can't get out of bed, what about doing some moves there? (The bed version of the F-It

Workout is there for you if you need ideas—see page 56.) In addition to the physical activity you'll get out of your more manageable alternative, you'll also be proving to yourself that exercise doesn't have to look and feel a certain way or unfold exactly as you intended.

Enlist outside support. Maybe what you really need is a benevolent external force. Someone you can turn to when you need a push—or a gentle nudge—into action. My mom still loves running, but like a lot of us, she's not suffering from an overabundance of energy and enthusiasm. Sometimes I get a text from her that says "I'm dressed. Just tell me to get out the door." Then I tell her to get it over with and think about how glad she'll be when she's done and then she does and then she is.

And if you don't have anyone in your life who can fill that role, maybe I can help.

Ready?

Get it over with! Picture how glad/relieved you'll be when it's over and you don't have to think about it anymore!

THE F-IT WORKOUT

I've put together this workout for days when you're low on motivation, nothing else is clicking, and you just want someone to tell you what to do. This collection of basic, practical moves is designed to touch on all of your major muscle groups, move your body in every direction, and give you a little taste of strength, cardio, and mobility. Instead of a full body blast, consider this a full body friendly nudge.

As always, the numbers here are suggestions, not hard rules. Feel free to adjust them to better suit your needs. You can either plow right through these exercises or take a short break (say 30 seconds to 1 minute, or whatever feels right) between each one.

And if this is still too much to handle, there's a variation you can do in bed on page 60.

---

1 | **TORSO TWISTS:** 1 minute or 30 reps per side

Stand with your feet hip distance apart. Bend your arms and hold them at shoulder height, parallel to the floor. Rotate your upper body from side to side.

---

2 | **STANDING SIDE BENDS:**
1 minute or 15 reps per side

Still standing with your feet hip distance apart, reach your right arm in the air over your head and bend your upper body to the left. (Be careful not to bend forward or back at the waist. If it helps, imagine that you're in between two panes of glass.) Return to center. Repeat on the opposite side.

---

3 | **BUTT KICKERS:** 1 minute or 30 reps per leg

March or jog in place while kicking your heels toward your butt.

4   HIGH KNEES: 1 minute or 30 reps per leg

March or jog in place while lifting your knees to about hip height. (If it helps you focus, hold your hands out in front of you just below waist level and try to hit your hands with your knees as you march.)

5   SHOULDER CIRCLES:
30 seconds or 20 reps in each direction

Stand with your feet hip distance apart and reach your arms out in front of you. Keeping a soft bend in your elbows (this prevents you from hyperextending your arms during the movement) and maintaining a moderate pace, circle both arms backward, down, and around to the starting position. When you've finished your reps, repeat in the opposite direction.

6   SQUATS: 1 minute or 15 reps

Stand with your feet slightly wider than hip distance apart and your toes slightly turned out. Keeping a nice, tall posture (don't round your back and look down), shift your hips back and start to lower them like you're sitting down in a chair. Pause when your thighs are parallel to the floor, and then return to the starting position with control.

7   ONE-LEGGED DEADLIFTS:
30 seconds or 8 reps per leg

Balance on your right foot. Keeping your back and your left leg straight, slowly bend forward until your torso and left leg are parallel to the floor. Slowly return to the starting position. When you've finished your reps, switch legs. (If you need help with balance, you can place both of your hands on the back of a chair in front of you, or your left hand on the back of a chair to your left, while doing this one. If that's still not working for you, you can also do the movement with both feet planted on the floor, bending at the torso.)

8 SHOULDER RETRACTIONS (OR A SEXIER NAME OF YOUR OWN CREATION THAT YOU LIKE MORE):
1 minute or 15 reps

Grab a towel, yoga strap, or other piece of fabric (T-shirt, etc.), and pull it taut between your hands around waist level. With your hands slightly wider than shoulder distance apart, raise the fabric until it and your arms are parallel to the floor. Keep that same amount of tension in the fabric as you slowly glide your shoulder blades together and gently squeeze. Slowly relax your shoulder blades and return to the starting position.

9 WALL PUSH-UPS: 1 minute or 15 reps

Stand in front of a wall. Place your palms on the wall, about shoulder distance apart and slightly lower than shoulder height. Look toward the wall, straighten your arms, and come up on your toes. Adjust as necessary until you feel comfortable and ready to do push-ups from that position. Gently engage your core, maintain good posture, and slowly lower your chest toward the wall, and then push yourself back to the starting position. (You can do these from your knees or from your feet on the ground if you want and can handle the extra challenge, but you don't *need* to. Wall push-ups are legit!)

10 SLOW MOUNTAIN CLIMBERS: 30 seconds or 10 reps per side

Get into a plank position with your hands on the floor (or on the wall if you're not feeling up to a full plank). Place your feet hip distance apart and your hands shoulder width apart. Engage your core and glutes to maintain a safe and solid posture that doesn't put too much pressure on your lower back. Keeping that core engagement, slowly draw one knee toward your chest, and return it to the starting position. Repeat with the opposite knee to complete 1 repetition.

11 SHADOWBOXING: 1 minute or 60 punches

Have some fun with this one. Throw whatever jabs, crosses, hooks, and uppercuts (and knees and kicks if you're so inclined) that you want for the allotted reps or time. And if you don't know what those are or how to do them "properly," just start punching the air however you feel like it.

12 ROLL DOWNS: 30 seconds or 5 reps

Stand with your legs hip distance apart. Keeping your lower body in place, nod your head and slowly roll your spine down one vertebra at a time until the crown of your head is reaching toward the floor. Take a deep breath down here and then slowly roll back up again. Repeat.

THE F-IT WORKOUT (IN BED)

1   **SPINE TWISTS:** 1 minute or 30 reps

Lie flat on your back and stretch your arms out to your sides. Bend your knees and place your feet on the bed about 6 inches from your butt. Turn your head to the left and slowly lower your knees to the right. Repeat on the opposite side to complete 1 repetition.

2   **SIDE BENDS TOE TOUCHES:** 1 minute or 20 reps per side

Still with your knees bent and feet flat on the bed, bring your arms down to your sides. Keeping your head and torso in contact with the mattress, bend at your waist to reach your right fingertips toward your right ankle. Switch sides to complete 1 repetition.

3   **BUTT KICKERS:** 1 minute or 30 reps per leg

Roll onto your stomach and rest your forehead on your hands. Gently engage your abs (think of drawing your belly button a little closer to your spine) to support your lower back in this position. Then alternate kicking your heels toward your butt.

4   **KNEE RAISES:** 1 minute or 20 reps per leg

Roll onto your back. Straighten your left leg, and bend your right knee and gently pull it toward your chest. Pause, then gently release the leg and switch sides.

5 SHOULDER CIRCLES:
1 minute or 15 reps in each direction

Still on your back, bend both knees, place your feet on the bed, and lay your arms along your sides. Lift your arms up to point at the ceiling and then sweep them over your head, out to the sides, and back down again. Then switch directions: out to the sides, over your head, up to the ceiling, and down.

6 SHOULDER BRIDGES: 1 minute or 15 reps

On your back with knees bent, feet flat, and arms at your sides, engage your butt and lift your hips off the bed. Then slowly lower yourself back to the starting position.

7 LEG PRESSES:
30 seconds on each leg or 10 reps per leg

You will need a towel, blanket, shirt, or other piece of fabric for this exercise. Still lying on your back, place your right foot in the middle of the towel, bend your knee, and draw your knee toward your chest. Grab the ends of the fabric and pull until there's a small amount of tension in it. Straighten your left leg. Keep pulling gently on the fabric to give yourself a little resistance while you push your right foot toward the ceiling and straighten that leg. (Your arms can move a little with the movement. You don't have to hold on for dear life and rip the fabric with your strong quads. You're just trying to give yourself a little bit of resistance here.) Slowly return to the starting position and repeat. Then switch legs.

8   SEATED SHOULDER RETRACTIONS (OR A SEXIER NAME OF YOUR OWN CREATION THAT YOU LIKE MORE): 1 minute or 15 reps

Sit up and either cross your legs, bend your knees, or straighten them in front of you, whatever's most comfortable. Grab your piece of fabric again and pull it tight between your hands. With your hands slightly wider than shoulder distance, raise the fabric until it and your arms are parallel to the floor. Keep the same amount of tension in the fabric as you slowly glide your shoulder blades together and gently squeeze. Slowly relax your shoulder blades and return to the starting position. (You can also try these while lying down if you don't feel like sitting up.)

9   OVERHEAD PRESS: 1 minute or 15 reps

Lie on your back with knees bent and feet flat on the bed. Grab the fabric as you did in #8 and engage your core so that you don't arch your back during the movement. Then reach your arms over your head so that your fists are pointing toward the ceiling. Then return to the starting position.

10   DEAD BUGS: 1 minute or 10 reps per side

Still lying on your back, pull your belly button toward your spine until your lower back comes into contact with the mattress. Bend your knees and lift your legs until your knees are directly above your hips and your shins are parallel to the bed. Reach your arms up straight, pointing your fingertips to the ceiling. Keeping your lower back in contact with the mattress, reach your right arm over your head and straighten your left leg out at a 45-degree angle. Return to the starting position and switch sides.

11 | BARREL ROLLS: 1 minute or 20 rolls per side

Lie on your back in the middle of the bed with your legs straight and your arms reaching overhead. Roll to one side and then to the other.

12 | CORPSE POSE: 1 minute or until you're bored

Lie flat on your back with your arms and legs extended and just hang out like that for a while.

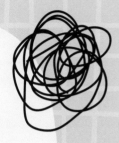

- THREE -

THAT COUNTS

Why your workout habits don't
need to be as formal, consistent,
extensive, or typical as you think
they do

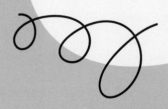

Thankfully, the Reagan-era slogan "No pain, no gain" is on its way out. Everyone except the most merciless old-school coaches is beginning to realize that the motto is harmful, ultimately counterproductive, and scientifically bullshit. Pain is your body's way of telling you that something is wrong. Pushing yourself to that level of suffering isn't better for you—plus it's a good way to get hurt, which in fact puts you at a loss. But the all-or-nothing thinking that gave us a generation of muscle tees with bad slogans and worse graphic design is still with us. And its insidious influence on our concept of fitness is everywhere.

If it's not hard or heavy enough, do you even lift, bro? If it's not fast enough, long enough, or perfect enough, why even bother? If it's not performed in the right venue, with the right equipment, and as exactly as suggested, you're only cheating yourself. And if it too closely resembles something you might do for fun, well, does it *really* count?

This attitude has influenced us in not one but two terrible ways. First, it's conditioned us to believe that nothing short of pushing yourself to (and beyond) your breaking point is good enough, or even a meaningful effort. Secondly, it's fostered a fitness industry in which exercise is something people sell—which means convincing customers they're getting their money's worth, which often means exploiting those very ideas about how you're only pushing yourself hard enough if you're pushing yourself too hard. (On the flip side, trainers who try to keep their workouts responsible, sustainable, and achievable sometimes lose customers who think they should be suffering. I've had clients tell me that because they could move without too much pain the next day, they felt they were wasting their money.)

Our bodies don't keep score like that, though. Your muscles aren't going to void the physical benefits of your first nine reps if you can't safely execute a tenth one. Your cardiovascular system isn't going to refuse to adapt if you prefer to take it on walks instead of runs. Your heart rate doesn't know the difference between a dance floor and an aerobics studio. And as we've established, your mind and your mood will probably benefit from anything you can manage to do. It all adds up. It all counts.

Exercise isn't a complete free-for-all, but most of the rules and guidelines that exist are far more flexible than we've been led to believe. The only ones I'd consider universal are about safety, i.e., do this exercise this way so that you don't hurt yourself or risk long-term issues. Everything else depends on the person and their situation. A competitive athlete needs to follow specific training protocols to achieve their peak performance. Someone who wants a six-pack is going to need to perform certain moves, follow a certain diet, and, let's face it, have a certain genetic predisposition.

For the kind of goals that this book is addressing, though? Our options are almost limitless. The only hard rule here is don't do anything that harms you—physically *or* mentally.

YOU GOTTA WANT IT (AND YOU CAN)

Don't worry about what you *should* do. There's no definitive answer to that, anyway.

There is no perfect exercise. There's no one-size-fits-all solution that will give everyone a clear mind and quarter-bouncing glutes if only they force themselves through the activity X minutes X times per week. There's not even one great option that can be easily modified to suit most populations and make them all feel pretty good. The fitness world is constantly searching for that holy grail, and there are always people in that world who will act like they've found it. But even their answers change with time. In the 1980s and early 1990s, high-impact aerobics was the be-all and end-all. When that generation of instructors started realizing the long-term impact of all of those classes on their joints, they pivoted to mind-body workouts like yoga and Pilates and lower-impact cardio like Spinning. Then, as far as I can tell, my generation of trainers got bored and threw everything and everyone into bootcamps, CrossFit, and high-intensity interval training. Now we're starting to see the fallout of some of those methods.

The good news is that fitness keeps changing because our understanding of it keeps changing and growing. We learn more about the human body and the science of exercise, and then we apply it. The middling news is that this new information is always filtered through an individual's interpretations and biases—and sometimes through their need to spin it into hot new workouts and products—which leaves us with mixed results. There's valuable wisdom and exercise ideas in almost all of these trends, but they all have their faults, too. (If you ever get frustrated with your efforts to find something that works for you, just remember: the experts are still figuring their stuff out, too.)

Instead of *should*, think about what you *want* to do and what you might enjoy trying. If your brain isn't willing to go so far as enjoyment or desire at the moment, you can also aim for what you'd hate the least.

The best workout is one you can do. It's one you won't dread, too, because what's the sense of making yourself miserable before and during a training session when the whole purpose of doing it is to feel less bad? This is true regardless of what activity you choose. For example, say there *was* some ideal workout that everyone agreed was the one you "should" do—but all you could manage to do was five minutes of log rolls back and forth in bed. (It's a warm-up exercise if you do it on a martial arts mat, so it counts on a mattress, too.) Those five minutes of rolling will be so much more beneficial to you than the zero minutes of that other workout that didn't end up happening. Based on that simple calculation alone, it's already the better choice.

But that's not all. You will probably spend less time and mental energy having to psych yourself up to do your five-minute roll than you would having to force yourself to do that other thing. And at the end of those five minutes, you'll get to feel a sense of accomplishment. Or at least a sense of relief.

So on one hand, you have a hypothetical perfect workout that, for whatever reason, you can't or won't do. It takes significant time and mental energy to attempt and makes you feel like crap if you don't go through with it, which puts more pressure on any future attempts. That experience only leaves with you new sources of stress and pain and little to no actual exercise.

On the other hand, you have a good-enough workout that you can and probably will do. You can start and finish it with relatively little mental effort, and it might just make you feel OK about yourself when you can do it—which makes the next time a little less daunting. Your brain cannot use this as proof that you fail at everything and you suck. The experience leaves you with a new exercise, has somewhere between a neutral and good impact on your life, and could lead to the start of a routine.

Which one sounds like the better workout now?

You can apply this general equation to any supposedly great workout that you're dreading. Starting and finishing an exercise like that is likely going to require a much higher mental load. Plus you'll need to be extra careful during it, because performing intense exercise while tired or checked out comes with a higher risk of injury. You might feel great or wretched afterward. It might become easier and more enjoyable in time, or it could always be a slog and a source of dread. It might lead to genuinely amazing changes in your life, or it could leave you injured and feeling worse. It all depends on you, your circumstances, and how you want to navigate your wretched but manageable workout. There might be days when you feel like dealing with all of the above, and there will definitely be days when you don't.

But an exercise that you can manage to do and want to do most of the time is always going to be better than an exercise you have to force yourself into, perform wrong because you're grumpy, or never do at all. You can probably find one of these that's a little more intensive than barrel rolling, but so what if it's not? Rolling from side to side isn't going to contribute to strength, conditioning, or even mental functioning as much as doing a more intensive workout—but it will help a lot more than *not* doing one, and sometimes that's the choice at hand.

FORGET THE FORMULA

If you've ever had a personal training session, attended a fitness class, or watched a video, you might have noticed that most workouts follow the same general formula. There's a warm-up. Then there's some form of cardio and strength training. (The percentage of each depends on the style, but there's almost always a mix of the two.) Maybe there's a special abs section. Finally, there's the cooldown.

This isn't a terrible format, and there's nothing nefarious behind its development. Although the exact wording and classification can vary between sources, most fitness and wellness authorities consider strength, muscular endurance, cardiovascular fitness, body composition, and flexibility the major health-related components of fitness. Most general-audience workouts are designed to touch on all of these.

This basic template is good for its audience: people with general fitness goals who have the motivation and executive function to enable them to hire a trainer, sign up for classes, or source a video and equipment to pursue and follow through on regular exercise. If you've got that much going for you, it doesn't matter so much if you like cardio more than strength, or find warm-ups boring, or whatever. You can just grumble through whatever chunk of the workout you don't love. When everything involved in getting started—or considering getting started—is already a barrier, though, that chunk can be far more than an unpleasant task. It could become a dealbreaker.

All the major components of fitness—strength, muscular endurance, cardiovascular fitness, and flexibility—have value. In an ideal situation, you could benefit from a program that addresses them all. If you find something that works for you now, there's a good chance you'll hit a point where it will be useful to consider including different aspects of fitness in your routine. But if you're not in an ideal situation right now, not a single one of those components is so crucial that it's worth risking what little motivation and self-confidence you have. Do what you can. Do what you want to do. And you can worry about the rest later, if you need to at all.

If you hate cardio, you don't have to do cardio. If it's going to stand between you and the rest of a perfectly good workout, then skip it. Or come up with a substitute that pleases you. The same goes for strength training. Stretching, too. Nothing in fitness is universal or irreplaceable. Your workout doesn't instantly become inferior or a waste of time because you didn't include a specific kind of exercise. Don't think of such an absence as a deficit in your routine. Focus on all of the things you might try—and all of the benefits that could result from trying them—if you give yourself permission to take the loathsome thing(s) off your plate.

You can always come back to it later. Once you find a workout you don't hate, and you start to experience exercise as something other than a source of aggravation, guilt, pain, and/or failure, you might find yourself developing a new curiosity for other forms of it. Or you might discover a new side to something you don't love that makes it worth your time and effort. I know a runner who always hated weights and could never find a strength program that she wanted to stick with for more than a few sessions. While sidelined with a flare-up of an old injury, though, she decided to try a weight-lifting routine that was geared toward injury prevention. After a few months, she started to notice an improvement not just with her injury but in her running overall. She still doesn't love the weights, but she appreciates how they contribute to something she does love—which makes them genuinely useful to her. Of course, it's possible that you will always hate something and never find a point to it, and that's perfectly fine, too. You can spend the rest of your life happily moving your body in other ways.

BUST THIS MYTH:
"NEVER SKIP LEG DAY"

Originally, the concept of leg day was almost entirely contained to serious lifting and bodybuilding communities. Basically, the body parts that were most celebrated in those fitness circles (pecs, delts, abs, etc.) are developed through upper-body training. Depending on context, the idea of skipping leg day might be a taunt about aesthetics (dudes with built upper bodies and no lower-body muscles wind up looking like really jacked cobras), or a gentle reminder to seek more balance in your workouts.

For a general audience, "never skip leg day" is mostly a scold about laziness. Many people—myself included—find lower body workouts more challenging and the post-workout recovery period more unpleasant. The delayed onset muscle stiffness I get from a leg day workout lasts almost twice as long as the one I get from upper-body training. But honestly, even people who love training their lower bodies think leg day kind of sucks sometimes. And most of us are not going to get to the point where doing too few squats makes us dangerously unbalanced.

Lower-body workouts can be great—strong glutes, quads, hamstrings, and calves likely make you springier and faster. But lower-body weight training isn't for everyone, and it doesn't have to be.

If you hate squats, don't do them! If deadlifts bore you to tears, trade them for something that doesn't. If lunges make you feel unstable and nervous, scrap them. You don't have to conform to this (or any) exercise ideal. Exercise needs to make itself valuable to you. Making it a regular part of your life is not about what you need to force yourself to do every time. It's about finding the thing you don't always want to skip.

(One caveat: whatever you end up doing or not doing, I strongly recommend including a warm-up and cooldown. I'm not going to say that you have to do these things. If the very thought of them is making you start to shut down, then skip them, too. But they actually are as good as fitness nerds insist they are. Gradually ramping up to your main workout prepares your mind and body for the task and reduces your risk of exhaustion and injury. Ramping down at the end eases you back into normal life activity, better prepares you to face the next workout, and lowers your risk of long-term injury. Almost everyone will benefit from adding an intro and outro to their physical activities. It doesn't have to be a formalized process, either. If traditional warm-up and cooldown routines are a turnoff, you can walk for five minutes, or do a less intense version of an exercise you don't hate. Or a few minutes of general full-body flailing while whining that you don't love this but you guess it has a purpose.)

LET'S GET WEIRD

Your workout doesn't have to include traditional exercises that are designed to address specific components of fitness. It doesn't have to look like a traditional workout at all. There's a whole world beyond gyms, studios, tracks, and mats, and there are countless ways to move your body. Just because something is also a hobby, a social event, or an activity you do alone to amuse yourself doesn't mean that it's not exercise. It all counts, too. (I didn't mean "amuse yourself alone" like *that*, but you're free to run with it if you want. It gets the heart rate up, after all.)

In no particular order, here's a brief sampling of unconventional exercises you can try. Some require training or equipment that you might not have access to if there aren't classes in your area, but others you can do just with a friend or even alone.

AERIAL SILKS

Aerial gymnastics, an art form in which a performer executes acrobatic moves while suspended from one or two pieces of fabric, was first popularized by Cirque du Soleil in the 1990s and 2000s. Since then, it's been adapted for a wide range of skill levels and disciplines. Aerial classes in acrobatics, yoga, and Pilates are now offered all over the world.

Aerial skills are particularly good for developing upper-body and core strength and endurance. You might be surprised at the level of cardiovascular endurance that you'll develop with regular training, too, not to mention the boost you'll see in secondary fitness components such as balance and coordination. This kind of workout is a great option for people looking for a new source of artistic expression, people who want to do more mind-body work but feel uninspired by more common mat-based exercises, and anyone who wants to swoosh around and try to recapture the childhood rush of swinging around on playground equipment.

REBOUNDING

You know those cool-looking mini trampolines? Rebounding is the style of aerobic workout that's been developed for them. Rebounding is a good form of low-impact cardio and can improve core and lower-body muscular endurance, balance, coordination, and agility. Mini rebounding trampolines are also relatively affordable (you can get a decent model for around $50) and they don't take up a lot of space, which makes them an ideal home exercise option. And if you don't feel up to an entire workout, you can always pull out your trampoline and do some unstructured jumping up and down for a quick rush.

HEMA

Broadly speaking, historical European martial arts (HEMA) refers to a category of martial arts of European origin that have either died out or evolved into modern sports such as fencing. The HEMA community is dedicated to reviving these martial arts through research, practice, and swords. HEMA's collaborative learning environment, strong online presence, and clubs across North America and Europe make it a great option for anyone motivated and encouraged by community participation. The swords make it a good choice for anyone who finds "normal" exercise boring, or anyone who's ever dreamed of playing with a sword. And the martial arts are an excellent way to develop cardio, full-body muscular endurance, coordination, agility, balance, speed, reaction time, and power.

ROLLER SKATING

In addition to giving you an aura of retro cool, roller skating in general improves cardiovascular power and endurance, balance, speed, and core and lower-body strength. Depending on what you do in your skates, you might also work on your agility, reaction time, and stress relief. A pair of skates opens up a bunch of potentially fun new activities, too. You can skate outside or at a rink. You can pursue artistic roller skating if you're into expression or aggressive inline skating if you're into tricks. If teamwork and contact sports appeal to you, roller derby is still going strong in many North American cities. If you like the idea of roller skating but hate being perceived, you can try it from home provided you have space and the right flooring. A friend of mine taught herself to skate in the kitchen of her one-bedroom apartment during the COVID-19 pandemic.

PILLOW FIGHTING

As a former professional pillow fighter, I can assure you that swinging those things was one of the most challenging and cathartic workouts I've ever done. As far as I know, you can't go pro anymore, but try it alone or with a friend. It's a fun way to blow off steam and an excellent way to sneak in some cardio and core work.

If you can find a willing participant, head to a space where you can responsibly swing a pair of pillows (I recommend fiberfill) and go at each other for one- or two-minute rounds. If not, try solo drills: Hold a pillow overhead in both hands and hit the ground as hard as possible. Then hold it over one shoulder, either double- or single-handed, and swing it toward the ground on the opposite side. Repeated on the other side. Then alternate. You can also mount a pillow and do MMA-style ground-and-pound drills on it. Hammer fists drills, where you repeatedly strike the pillow with the bottoms of your fists, are especially fun. If the structure doesn't appeal to you, you can always freestyle.

RETRO EXERCISE VIDEOS

Not everything in workout videos from the 1980s and 1990s has aged well. (The speed and lack of control on some of those original Jane Fonda leg lifts is alarming.) But I suspect the main reason they've gained a reputation for being outdated, unserious, and cringey is because they made exercise accessible and welcoming to people who couldn't or wouldn't set foot in a gym. Overly stern gatekeeping types didn't like that, so they dismissed and mocked them. And, for some reason, a lot of us started believing the bullies.

But there's little in most of these old videos, most of which you can find streaming online, that can't be easily modified to suit our current knowledge of exercise and your current goals. (If you slow down those Fonda leg lifts so that you're moving within your hip's range of motion and not using your

SWEATING TO THE OLDIES

If the retro exercise tape idea sounds good to you, but you're not sure where to start, here are some of my favorites to get you going. You'll probably be able to find hard copies of most of these titles online or at a thrift store if you're a collector. But they're all through streaming services and YouTube if you're not:

- *Richard Simmons's 5 Minute Workout with Attitude:* I'm pro-*Sweatin' to the Oldies* in general. Any title you can find from the series is worth checking out. I'm specifically suggesting this brief excerpt that's been posted on YouTube, though, because it's such a perfectly distilled dose of the Simmons experience. There's a lot going on in this clip. The workout is a nice little aerobics routine. Everything surrounding it is pure chaos. Some people are doing the choreography in workout clothes. Some are doing it in jeans and polo shirts. Others—including two women in club wear and high heels—appear to be making up their own moves as they go along. Oh, and all of this is happening in a fake mall. It's perfect for when you need a reminder that fitness doesn't have to be so bloody serious.

- *Step Reebok: The Video:* This one's another incredible mix of solid workout principles and bonkers set design. It switches things up enough to keep people interested but the exercises aren't so complex that rookies will tune out or give up. Higher impact moves such as jumps are introduced carefully and used in moderation. The entire vibe . . . well, I think they were going for a "Rhythm

Nation" vibe, but they wound up with something more like Apple's "1984" Superbowl ad. And I'm glad, because the video's dystopian aura is a welcome respite from the perkiness of almost every other video on the market.

- **Any Tae-Bo video:** Billy Blanks created something special with his Tae-Bo videos. He made a wide range of martial arts/combat sports techniques fun and accessible for people who would never have considered setting foot in a Taekwondo gym or boxing ring. And he made unbridled enthusiasm kind of cool. I also recommend the series of at-home Tae-Bo videos that Blanks made during the early days of the COVID-19 pandemic. If you've ever worried that exercising in your living space isn't "real" enough, seeing a fitness legend pushing his couch back and exercising on his living room rug will set you straight.

- **Do It Debbie's Way:** There are a number of things I could say to sell Hollywood legend Debbie Reynolds's foray into beginner aerobics. The set features Roman columns, a chandelier, and Debbie's name in lights! She admits that she wouldn't be doing any of this if she'd had more recent success! Shelley Winters rolls around in the background and gossips the whole time! But nothing I could say would capture this video's spirit half as well as this excerpt from Reynolds' rambling introduction: "I never really thought I was going to do a program like this, but you know what happened to me? I went out and I bought all of these other tapes, which are excellent, but I found that I really couldn't keep up with them. Well, maybe I didn't want to keep up with them because they're really fast." It truly is the perfect exercise video for when you just want to lie down.

waist to fling your leg overhead, you'll end up with a very effective butt move.) And lots of these videos are a fun change of pace from more modern workout trends and attitudes. Besides, what's more cringe: an earnest instructor in outdated fitness gear who wants you to have fun while doing low-impact moves, or some gym bro getting huffy because people might have fun dancing along instead of lifting?

SOLO DANCE PARTY

Put on a song and do whatever you want to it. Repeat as necessary. It's a solid source of cardio and stress relief. Depending on what kind of moves you're into, this might end up being a strength workout, too.

EXERCISE IS EVERYWHERE

Your workout doesn't *have* to look like a separate activity at all, though. If even the "fun" exercises feel insurmountable, keep in mind that they're just a step or two beyond what you're already doing. The simple act of living your life involves all sorts of movements. Moving to and from places, even if just to the bathroom and back. Showers. Cooking. Dishes. Laundry. Tidying. Fidgeting. Tossing and turning. A general flailing of limbs and cursing the universe. And so much more. All of these activities recruit your muscles and cardiovascular system. They all add up. They count, too.

There are also a ton of smaller activities that you can randomly incorporate into your day if you can't stomach the idea of doing a whole workout at once. Here's a brief list of ways that you can incorporate movement into your downtime. It's the tip of the iceberg, but it should be enough to help you see your many options and maybe inspire you to come up with your own.

- Sitting down and standing up: Grab a chair and stand in front of it. Sit down. Stand up. Repeat as many times as you want. This functional and relatively unannoying squat alternative works your calves, quads, hamstrings, and glutes and comes with a built-in resting spot when you're done.

- Lying down and standing up: If you're looking for a full-body variation of the previous move, or if you just want to be more dramatic, you can take it to the floor. Lie down. You can spend some time cursing the world and/or declaring that this is where you belong if that's the kind of mood you're in. Then get yourself to a standing position by whatever means are most comfortable and functional for you. Repeat as many times as you want. This will work all of your major muscle groups and probably become a decent cardio challenge after the first few reps.

- One-minute dance party: If you don't have the time or energy for a longer dance party, you can always throw on a favorite song for a quick burst. You'll get a little cardio blast and an instant mood boost.

- HIIT (wHatever Intensity Interval Television): If you're watching a show on an actual TV station, pick a move and do it during the commercial breaks. If you're streaming, search online to see if anyone has invented a drinking game for your show. Pick a move or two and substitute them for the shots.

- Random shadowboxing: It's surprisingly fun to randomly punch (and kick, if you have the space and inclination) the air when you're alone or with understanding company. Depending on your mood, it could also be a satisfying stress reliever. And there's a reason why professional fighters continue to make it a part of their training: it's great for cardio, upper body, core, and coordination.

- Staying in bed: If you can't get out of bed for whatever reason, you can also do random movements there. Arm circles. Side leg lifts. Hip releases. Crunches and leg raises if you want to get fancy. You could attempt a plank if you're up to it. And there's always log rolls.

- Taking the stairs (if you want to!): I hate that "take the stairs" has become a sweeping, condescending suggestion aimed at anyone in the vicinity of any elevator or escalator. Walking up a floor or two when you're already moving from one place to another is a good way to add a little extra oomph to your daily movements, but it isn't and shouldn't have to be for everyone. It should be a choice, not an imperative! If you are able to and you want to, try a flight or two from time to time. If it goes well, that's awesome. Please don't be a dick about it.

Finally, you can also take steps to make your workout more enjoyable. And I don't just mean in a fitness-nerd way where you find yourself realizing what a blast it is to do a bunch of burpees one day. I mean incorporating stuff that you do for fun in your downtime into your fitness time. Put on a podcast, audiobook, or TV show while you work out. Map out a walk or a run that ends at your favorite coffee shop, and cool down by ordering a post-workout recovery treat and strolling home. Schedule a play date with a like-minded friend, or call someone who's up for chatting while you get your reps or mileage in. If you're never going to love the workout itself, build something into the workout that you will look forward to.

You don't have to suffer to get something out of your workouts. You don't have to struggle mentally or physically before, during, or after. In fact, for our purposes, you'll benefit more from physical activities that don't make your life worse in any way.

In other words: when you eliminate the pains, that's when you start to gain.

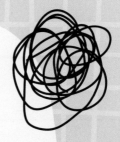

– FOUR –

BREAK IT UP

How to build a modular workout
that adapts to your energy level

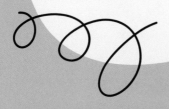

Imagine you're a competitive weight lifter. (Yeah, I realize it's kind of out there given the entire premise of the book, but I promise I'm going somewhere with this.) The specifics of your training would vary depending on who you were working with and what training tables they were using. But in general terms, if you were lifting for power, you would be doing very heavy lifts for one or two reps at a time and resting for up to five minutes before doing it again.

If you were a long-distance runner, your training plan would include runs that focused on distance but also runs that focused on pace, hill work, cross-training, and rest.

If you were an amateur boxer, you would spar, but you'd also have separate training dedicated to technique, power, and cardio. And then you'd compete in a set number of timed rounds with a minute of rest in between.

Everything in fitness and athletics is broken up in some way. Every workout or training session is a collection of pieces that have been assembled to address an individual's needs and goals. This is how all serious exercisers, from recreational fitness buffs to professional athletes, approach physical activity.

This is exactly what you'll be doing if you choose to break your workout into the smallest pieces possible. It's not taking the easy way out or babying yourself. It is serious-business training with classic, tried-and-true methods. It's what powerlifters, marathoners, and heavyweight champs do.

WHY YOU SHOULD BREAK UP YOUR WORKOUTS

The short answer is so you can actually do them. (And not seriously hurt yourself in the process.)

To go back to my examples, a powerlifter definitionally cannot lift their one-rep maximum—the most weight they are physically capable of lifting—more than once. That's why it's called a *one-rep* maximum. A distance runner can't run their full race distance at goal pace every time they go out. (The marathon's origin story, the legend of Pheidippides, is about a man who *dies of exhaustion* after running a phenomenal distance.) Few boxers would survive for more than a couple of rounds if all they did was whale on each other with no time limit every time they went to the gym. In each case, these athletes would also be putting themselves at a drastically higher risk of injury and illness—which, in addition to being terrible in its own right, would put their goals even further out of reach. Worst-case scenario, attempting to do too much too hard could literally kill them.

In order to avoid this entire spectrum of terrible outcomes, coaches, trainers, recreational athletes, and fitness enthusiasts take the amount of activity that would be impossible or extremely unwise to tackle all at once and break it down into chunks that can be handled safely and effectively. So the powerlifter lifts an amount that will sufficiently challenge them and develop their strength and explosive power. Then they'll pause to allow their body to rest and their mind to prepare for the next part, and repeat for a responsible number of sets and lifts. The runner takes on smaller distances at various paces and saves the maximum effort for a responsible number of race days per year. Recreational runners may break down their races into intervals of walking and running, too. The boxer prepares by sparring at lower intensities and engaging in other forms of low- and no-contact training to fine-tune their game. They compete in short, powerful bursts interspersed with regular periods of mandated inactivity that enable them to rest, refocus, and rehydrate.

In terms of the kind of goals we're focusing on in this book, we are looking for tasks that are physically and mentally achievable. And while the amounts of exercise we're looking at are extremely unlikely to put you at serious risk of injury or literal death in excess, you're also going to want to avoid amounts of exercise that make you *feel* like death.

If you are depressed, anxious, burned out, or otherwise at odds with the act of existing and everything you're supposed to do to maintain your existence, taking on too much can overload *and* overwhelm you. So, like professional athletes, you could strongly benefit from breaking your workout down into components that you can safely finish without risking injury and overtraining. But you also need to break it down into pieces that you can safely *start*, without risking demoralization and self-reproach and heightened levels of anticipatory anxiety and wondering why you should even bother.

Once you've found an amount of exercise that your mind and body are prepared to take without too much consternation, you can start to look at ways you can assemble your manageable pieces into modular workouts. But first, you have to figure out what those pieces are.

HOW TO KNOW IF YOU'RE DOING ENOUGH

If you're as incapable of extending yourself grace as I am, you might find yourself struggling with the suggestion that your mental state should factor into this calculation. If you can physically do X amount of an exercise then surely you should just suck it up, stop being such a pathetic baby, and do X all at once, right?

No.

If you can physically do X but you find yourself putting it off or avoiding it entirely, guess what? X is officially more than you can do right now. Something you can theoretically do but can't actually do is *something you can't do*. And it's better to do a little less—or a lot less—than your theoretical maximum if the alternative is doing *nothing* because you're so upset over not doing *more*. Besides, if one of your workout goals is to improve your mental state, then your mental state should factor into your workout plans.

As for how small you can make your digestible chunks of exercise, the answer is: as small as they need to be to get you started. No caveats. Keep whittling away at the amount of exercise you're attempting until "I can't do this" or "I'm not effing doing this" turns into "fine, I guess I'll do this."

Is one wall push-up enough? If the thought of two wall push-ups is already way too much for you, let alone the thought of a push-up from your knees or your feet, then yes. That's where you start.

If you do your one wall push-up and it feels all right, you can try a second one. Or you can take a short break and then do another one. And another one, if you're up for it. You can turn around and add a wall angel for what gym nerds would call a superset. (Stand with your hips, upper back, and the back of your head pressed against a wall. Lift your arms up like you're doing the Y in YMCA and press your forearms and the backs of your hands against the wall, too. Keeping all of those things in contact with the wall, slowly glide your elbows down until the Y becomes a W. Then slowly return to the Y.) Or step back and add a squat. Try another set or two if you're up for that. Or do one push-up, decide you've had enough, and come back the next day feeling accomplished, refreshed, and ready to do it again. And again the day after that.

It's true that a single push-up of any variation is not a workout. You won't wake up with bulging pecs the morning after you've done it. But that push-up can be the foundation of a more enjoyable routine, and it can lead to a more rewarding relationship with physical movement. Which could lead to a clearer head. Which could also lead to pursuing a routine that could give you bulging pecs, if bulging pecs is what you decide you want. Slow progress that you can maintain and maybe even feel good about is exponentially better than pushing harder, feeling crappy, and potentially giving up.

How do you know if the pieces that you're assembling are enough for a workout? My philosophical answer is that enough is a nebulous concept and almost impossible to determine, particularly when every internal and external measure of sufficiency is influenced by a society that treats working yourself to the bone as the bare minimum. My practical answer is that it's likely going to take some trial and error to figure out what's right for you, but in general you're looking for an amount of exercise that makes you feel like you did something and like you could—and might even want to—do it again in the near future.

If you end up doing less than common fitness standards dictate, the worst that can happen is that your progress might be slower than what pushy exercise pros would consider normal. But almost every norm in fitness is messed up anyway, so what are you really missing out on? Why not take whatever time you need to build something better for yourself instead?

Choosing the blocks you're building with can be intimidating too—why are there so many types of push-up?—but, again, you can really be guided by how you feel. One type of push-up (or squat, or crunch) might work slightly different muscles and give you slightly different physical benefits from another, but that doesn't have to be the only factor in your decision, and it's not as important as establishing a routine that keeps you coming back. You can pick at random, or go for something that feels good when you do it, or that you think looks cool or hot. Or something that reminds you of another activity you enjoy. Or something tied to a good memory. Or literally anything else.

My favorite exercise is a "Hindu push-up," a variation that involves moving from downward dog to upward dog and back again. It's popular in martial arts training, which is where I picked it up. I enjoyed performing the move for its own sake—because I am a very cool person, I get excited about exercises that balance mobility and stability in the shoulder joint—but what made me fall in love with Hindu push-ups was their magical boundary-setting powers. I realized that doing a lot of them and doing them well during warm-ups made some gym bros back off or at least patronize me less. I have nothing left to prove now that I'm training alone, but I still get a nostalgic rush when I do them. I like what they do for my shoulders, but the real reason I keep doing them is because they make me feel assertive and powerful. And because they're kind of horny looking. "It looks horny and makes me feel powerful" is a perfectly good rationale for choosing a specific type of push-up out of the dozens of variations available.

BUILD A WORKOUT

Once you have your workout pieces, you can start to look at ways to put them together again. Like a Dadaist, 1990s industrial musician, Dr. Frankenstein, or whatever example of a reassembler you'd prefer.

There are a number of ways that you can do this, which I describe below. From a purely physical training perspective, they're all perfectly good for what we're trying to do. If you start to get into more specialized training, some of these methods will be better than others for your specific goal. Interval training is great for people who want to develop cardiovascular capacity and power, for example, but is suboptimal for muscle growth. If you choose to pursue more specific training goals in the future, you'll want to reevaluate your approach then.

But right now, all of these methods are equally capable of getting your mind to get your body where you want to go. So I'm going to focus on what kind of headspace each one is most suitable for.

(In each of these descriptions, I've included a short routine that I enjoy doing as an example, to give you an idea of how the same basic moves can be adapted for each workout format. You can try out this specific set of moves for yourself if you're interested, but you're just as free to never think about it again.)

COUNT IT

You do a move X times, you stop for Y amount of time, and then you repeat it for Z sets. You measure your work by counting the reps and sets. (Or you can hire or enlist someone to count for you.)

Reps and sets are most commonly associated with weight lifting, but you can apply the concept to other forms of exercise, too. Walk X laps of a track, rest for Y amount of time, repeat for Z sets. Hit a heavy bag with X jabs and X crosses, etc. You can combine moves for supersets: run X laps, do X lunges on each side. Rest and repeat your set (or superset) as desired. You can also switch up the number of reps per set or the amount of rest between sets. There are reasons why you might pick one of these variations over another in more specialized training, but for now, it's all about picking the one that's going to keep you interested and engaged.

The basic format of my sample routine is 5 of my beloved horny push-ups and 10 squats. The number of sets depends on my fitness level in general and my energy level on that day, but it's usually in the 4–6 range. So I do 5 push-ups and 10 squats, make sure nothing is hurting and my form is on point, then I go straight into my next 5 push-ups and 10 squats, and so on. As long as I feel relatively alive and I'm keeping everything moving safely, I keep going. If anything hurts or I completely run out of breath, I stop. If I notice that my form is starting to slip, or I feel fatigue creeping in, I'll aim for one last set.

I use this format when I want to have some control over my activity. Or when I need to feel like I have some control over any aspect of my life, if I'm being perfectly honest. You know exactly how much you need to do, how much you've done, and how much you still need to do. This can reduce anxiety of the unknown, ground you, and give you a sense of agency.

And if keeping track of reps and sets gets too confusing, you can also write them down as you go or use other counting aids. When my brain is a little foggy, I line up 6 of my cat's toys on one side of my mat and move 1 to the other side at the end of each set.

TIME IT

The basics of interval training can be applied to any form of physical activity and adjusted for any fitness level. You do a move or short series of moves for X amount of time, rest for Y amount of time, and repeat as necessary. You can use almost any ratio of work to rest time in this method. Ten minutes of movement to 1 minute of rest is great. But so is 5:1 or 1:1. You can also invert the ratio and rest for longer periods. A popular training interval is 1:2. If whole minutes sound like too much, choose intervals in seconds rather than minutes. Go with whatever works best for your body and brain.

When I don't feel like counting, I'll set a Tabata timer (20 seconds of work and 10 seconds of rest repeated 8 times) and alternate between push-up and squat sets for the work portion. If I still have the energy and drive to do so, I'll move on to another group of exercises using the same timer. If not, I'll cool down.

I use this format when I can't (or don't want to) focus or think too much. Turning on a timer and exercising until it goes off allows you to zone out for a while and worry about nothing more than whether you're moving safely. No keeping track. No keeping score. Just doing the thing until an outside force tells you it's time to stop. (You can also watch the clock, if that does it for you, although in my experience, that mostly leads to anxiety and misery.)

RANDOMIZE IT

In running, there's a loosely structured type of continuous interval training called fartleks. The name comes from the Swedish word meaning "speed play," and it's exactly what it says on the tin. You go for a run, and you play around with different speeds for different distances based on how you're feeling and what you want to accomplish that day. You can use specifically measured distances and times, like picking up your pace for 1 block or 1 minute, slowing down again for a set distance or time, and speeding up again. Or you

BUST THIS MYTH:
30 MINUTES A DAY

As far as fitness aphorisms go, this isn't the *worst*. As long as you're in the right headspace for it—and can do it without causing yourself harm—aiming for 30 minutes of moderate physical activity a day can be a low-pressure way to exercise for physical and mental health benefits. When it starts to feel more like an impossible standard than a gentle guideline, though, it becomes a problem.

There's no magic level of gains that kick in exactly at the half-hour mark. The amount of movement you do in a day isn't somehow negated if you don't hit it. Doing what you can and getting 5 minutes of activity in a day beats doing nothing because you know you can't do 30 so why bother. Doing 5 minutes of manageable and maybe even enjoyable movement a day, starting to build that into a routine, and possibly adding time to that routine as you progress beats 30 terrible minutes done under duress a few times that you can't maintain and eventually give up on. And focusing on what you can do beats worrying about what you should do. (By a lot. It's not even close.)

can go more free-form, like spotting a tree in the near distance and sprinting toward it, walking for a while and picking another tree, or listening to music and speeding up for some songs and returning to an easier starting pace for others.

Fartleks were designed for long-distance running, and they're most easily applied to forms of cardio in which you're propelling yourself forward (or mimicking forward propulsion on stationary equipment): running, cycling, inline skating, etc. But you can get creative and apply a fartlek-ish spirit to other forms of training, too. Put on a TV show and switch moves based on the location of each scene. Put on music and do one move for verses and another for the chorus (and another for the bridge if you're so inclined).

When I'm not in the mood to count sets or think about a timer, I put on a song—usually Skinny Puppy's "Assimilate (R23 Remix)" or Carly Rae Jepsen's "Run Away with Me," your mileage may vary—and do my 5 push-ups and 10 squats until it ends. If I'm up for more, I play another song and do another group of moves. This removes the pressure of keeping track of sets but is less likely to make me fixate than a timer. I have a general sense of where I am in the song and how much is left without getting hung up on the exact number of seconds.

In addition to the sense of agency that fartlek-style training can offer you, it also gently encourages you to pay attention to how your body is feeling and learn to adapt your training to that feedback. You start your workout, you take an assessment of how you're feeling and what you're up for, you pick a challenge based on that information, and you do it. Then you regroup, take another assessment, and base your next step on that.

CHRIS IT

I wasn't sure what to call this approach. *Deconstructed fartleks* and *microdose winging it* were contenders. But I've chosen to name it after a guy who came to all my classes when I was teaching indoor cycling, who inspired me to rethink how I structured my workouts and why.

Chris was always in class, but he never stuck around for a full one. He'd cycle for a couple of songs, get off the bike and wander out of the studio, return for a couple more, and then disappear again. I was confused at first, and maybe my ego was a little wounded. I'd worked hard to put together my workout plans. How dare he do his own thing!

But when I finally asked him what the hell he was doing, I quickly came around to his way of thinking. He was going to the weight room to squeeze some extra sets in. Which was weird, but also kind of brilliant. He was getting cardio and strength training in a way that clearly suited him. He wasn't hurting anyone, including himself, when he walked in and out of class. He wasn't disrupting anyone. He was just getting in the kind of workout he wanted to do in the space and time he had available.

I use the Chris method when I lack either the time, energy, or inclination to do anything resembling a bigger workout. I go about my day and I throw in a set of 5 push-ups and/or 10 squats when I can. Sometimes I'll write down the number of sets that I'm aiming to get done over the course of the day and cross them off as I go. But if that feels too serious or intimidating, I'll do them when I can and stop when I feel like I've done a satisfactory number or when I'm tired.

This approach comes in handy when you can't fit yourself into a traditional workout structure, but it's also helpful when you want to remind yourself that you don't have to! You can move when you want and how you want.

My only blanket suggestion here: If you're going to try this with medium- or high-intensity moves, you should do a quick warm-up first for injury prevention and generally making the hard move suck less for you.

If all of this is too free-form for you, I've included a template on page 96 that will enable you to assemble a basic modular workout. You can treat it like a prix fixe menu (or a Grand Slam, if you're more like me). The first thing to do is pick a tracking method from the options above. Then select a warmup, 3–5 exercises, and a cooldown. Do your warm-up, followed by your 3–5 exercises one time each. If you have the energy or want to responsibly push yourself more, you can repeat those exercises—and if you're still feeling good after that, you can do it again. Repeat as necessary. (Or don't! Doing one of each and moving on is perfectly fine too.) When you've finished your exercises, you'll do your cooldown.

Some of these choices will be pretty straightforward. If you're picking Time It, for example, you can do X minutes of warm-up, Y minute(s) of each exercise, and a Z-minute cooldown. Some will take a bit more creative logic. If you want to count but you also want to dance, you'll need to figure out a way to measure and counts units of dance. Maybe that means you do X full run-throughs of the "Single Ladies" chorus choreography, or maybe you tell yourself that you're going to wave your arms over your head X times and keep dancing until you hit that number. (You can also mix up your measurement styles. So you could, say, count your squats and then switch to timing your-self for the dance break portion.)

I'm going to leave it up to you to choose your X, Y, and Z—that is, the num-ber of repetitions or amount of time you want to do. I encourage you to apply everything we've covered in this chapter to figuring out what amount of each is right for you and where you're at right now.

You can modify or replace the suggested moves and play around with the timing as much as you want, or follow the recommendations included in the menu to the letter. Whatever works best for you.

BUILD YOUR OWN WORKOUT

1 ### PICK A MEASUREMENT:

- Count it (like reps and sets)
- Time it (like intervals or rounds)
- Randomize it (like fartleks)
- Chris it (like doing moves randomly throughout your day)

2 ### PICK A WARM-UP:

- Walking
- Light jogging
- Dynamic stretching (see page 111 for a basic routine)

3 ### PICK 3–5 EXERCISES:

You can go for an all-cardio, strength, or flexibility workout or mix it up.

Cardio
- Walking
- Jogging
- High-knee jogging
- Sprints
- Jumping jacks
- Steps (going up and down on single or multiple steps)
- Dancing (any style)
- Shadowboxing

Strength
- Squats
- Shoulder bridges

- Lunges
- Push-ups (on the wall, from the knees, or from the feet)
- Wall angels
- Back extensions
- Planks
- Side planks

Mobility

- High-knee march
- Heel kicks
- Standing hip circles (stand on one leg, bend the other knee, and draw circles from your hip joint in each direction)
- Torso twists
- Arm circles
- Cat/cow stretches

4 PICK A COOLDOWN:

- Marching on the spot
- Static stretching (see page 110 for a basic routine)
- Lying on the floor and gently full-body flailing

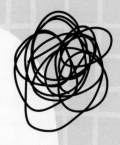

AROUND
THE BEND

Why flexibility is good for more
than just your schedule

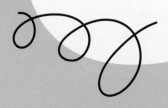

I f you don't feel up to doing a whole workout, what about a little bit of stretching?

You could even try some right now.

Sit or stand with a neutral posture. (Or lie down on your back with your legs either bent or straight if that's better for you.) Hold your book or reading device in front of you at eye level and gently lower your shoulders a little to ease some of the tension you're probably carrying in your trapezius muscles (which stretch over your neck, shoulders, and upper back). Don't forget to breathe.

Keeping your arms and torso in place, gently turn your head to the right, hold for a few seconds, and return to center. Do the same on the left side.

Now, keep looking forward, maintain that neutral posture, and tilt your head to the right. Think of gently reaching your ear toward your shoulder. (And make sure you're not lifting your shoulder toward your ear instead.) Hold it there for a few seconds. Then gently return to center. Now tilt your head to the left and hold. Come back to center.

Inhale and gently shrug your shoulders. Exhale to glide them back down. Inhale shrug, and exhale release. One more time. And relax.

Guess what? You just did an exercise. Yes, that counts, too.

If you're unconvinced, that's understandable. Stretching is rarely the flashiest workout option. It provides fewer opportunities for feelings of toughness and bragging rights. "Stretcher's high" isn't a thing. You don't hear people saying, "Bro! I just crushed that hip mobility sesh!" (Well, I do, but I am a nerd who hangs out with nerds.)

It doesn't help that almost everything we know about flexibility training—from how to do it to what it does and why—has changed in our lifetime. All that evolution and reassessment has left a lot of confusion and a touch of stigma in its wake. Maybe you've been given the impression that it's easy or a less serious form of exercise. Maybe you've been told that it doesn't work. Maybe all these messages have left you wondering if it's worth doing at all.

In my opinion, a lot of the scorn that flexibility training receives is unfair and the rest is often missing some nuance and perspective. Flexibility and mobility training don't have to be easy at all—unless you want them to be. There are some types of exercise with this focus that can seem unchallenging if you're not willing to take them seriously. There's a certain brand of gym bro that loves to half-ass their way through any workout that addresses flexibility and mobility and go on to dismiss the entire discipline when they don't think they get anything out of it. But I've never met anyone who has been open to instructions and willing to engage with the movements who felt like they weren't getting a legitimate workout.

As for whether or not stretching works, that all depends on what you're doing and what you want it to do for you.

The bad news is that the current science suggests that stretching doesn't do most of what we were told it did back in gym class—at least not the way we were taught to do it. Going straight from inactivity to pushing your muscles just past their comfort zone and holding them there for some number of seconds—or doing light cardio, stopping, and putting your slightly warmer muscles through this process—doesn't prevent injury or improve your performance during sports and exercise. And yanking cold muscles around until they hurt is a recipe for disaster. It's a miracle that our formative fitness years didn't hurt our bodies as regularly as they hurt our relationships with our bodies. (Fluidly moving your joints through their full range of motion, a.k.a. dynamic stretching, might help with performance and injury prevention, but currently there's no evidence to suggest that it's any more effective than other activities that gradually increase your activity level, encourage blood flow, and warm up muscle tissue. We'll learn more about dynamic stretching and range of motion later.)

Contrary to what we were once promised, basic stretching doesn't appear to change the shape of your muscles and is unlikely to transform your range of motion on its own, regardless of how well and faithfully you do it. It doesn't reduce the amount of muscle soreness you might experience after activity or provide more than the most temporary pain relief from knots and strains, either. Pushing too hard in your stretching can in fact lead to injuries and more pain.

But a regular basic stretching routine that involves responsibly pushing one's muscles as far as possible without feeling pain and holding that position for a period of time *does* seem to be able to change the way a person perceives the physical feeling and discomfort they experience during that activity. This increased stretch tolerance can and does lead to gradual long-term gains in flexibility, although those benefits probably aren't going to be as obvious, measurable, or as relatively fast as what you might get from strength training or cardio. In other words, stretching may not make you faster or more built, but it makes you better at stretching.

I suspect that this is what people are getting at when they say that stretching doesn't work or, my least favorite variation of this theme, "stretching doesn't work, it just feels good." Traditional stretching routines aren't performance enhancing and they don't lead to quick and obvious gains, so people who are focused on obvious gains think they must be worthless. This might be true for some people with specific goals. If you want to do the splits, have the game or workout of your life, avoid hurting yourself, and not feel delayed onset muscle soreness the next day, a little basic stretching will not do much for you. (It gives me no pleasure to inform you that I have never stumbled upon any pre- or postworkout tricks or supplements that do much to change my next-day soreness. I can only suffer and swear through it until the ache naturally fades.) Stretching shouldn't be your focus if you're primarily motivated by aesthetic and performance-based results.

But what if you want to do a moderate, low-pressure form of exercise that could gradually improve how you move and feel? That's not nothing. If you've ever been alienated from fitness—or your body—finding a way to move that feels pleasant and rewarding while you're doing it is a goddamned miracle. "It just feels good"? There's no "just" about that. (And there are methods of flexibility and mobility training that do a lot more than make you feel good. We'll get to that shortly.)

Stretching is actually a great place to start if your goals involve improving your mood and building a more rewarding relationship with movement. Even its limitations become assets in this context. You can't make a stretching workout about how hard you can go, what you can produce, or what it can make you look like. You *have* to focus on how it makes you feel and what that feeling does for you. If there's little to no hope of seeing big short-term gains from this type of exercise, then there's no point in pushing yourself too hard in pursuit of them. So you might as well focus on what makes you feel good during your stretches (or after you release them).

Paying attention to how you feel during a stretch isn't just an incidental benefit; it's also a fundamental part of the process. Stretching requires you to check in with your body. You move a muscle or a group of muscles as far as you can without feeling pain. (Mild discomfort is OK, but if it hurts, you've gone too far.) You hold that position for a number of seconds, reminding yourself to breathe. Then you gently release it and assess how your muscles feel in the aftermath. If something feels off at any point, you adjust accordingly. Some stretching programs will also encourage you to take your mental and emotional state into account. These can influence how you feel and move, so it's important to take them seriously and stretch in ways that will ease the physical stress your mental condition might be contributing to instead of exacerbating it. (I've often wondered if this is part of the reason that stretching receives so much negative attention in some fitness circles. A form of exercise that doesn't appeal to our capitalistic obsession with productivity *and* wants us to think about our feelings? How dare you!)

In addition to its general benefits, basic stretching has really useful applications for some of the issues we're addressing in this book. For anyone who has struggled with body awareness, a small routine that you can perform on your own provides a low-pressure and low-judgment opportunity to start figuring things out. It can be a source of stress relief when you're tense and have a grounding effect when you're anxious.

If you're in the throes of can't-get-out-of-bed depression, a stretch or two is something that you can perform with minimal effort that can give you a sense of accomplishment and a touch of physical relief. A little chest stretch after a long period of being curled in the fetal position makes me feel like a tiny fraction of the world's weight has been temporarily lifted.

WHO SHOULD USE CAUTION WHEN STRETCHING?

Stretching can be useful for a wide range of people, but there's no exercise that is healthy and beneficial for every single person on earth, and this is no exception.

If you are recovering from an injury or surgery, you should consult with your doctor or physical therapist to see which exercises, if any, are safe for you to attempt in your current condition.

If you are hypermobile in certain joints, you'll have to be careful and thoughtful about how you train the muscles that cross them. At best, stretching them won't feel like anything. At worst, it could hurt you and exacerbate problems you have in that area. Exercises that focus on developing a balance of stability and mobility in your joints might be a better option for you. I would recommend checking in with a doctor or movement specialist to get a better idea of your options. (I find Pilates schools that have incorporated rehab and PT influences to be a good source of this kind of training, but that's not all that's out there.)

People with conditions that affect your connective tissues, such as Ehlers-Danlos syndrome (EDS), will need to approach any kind of flexibility training with extreme caution. It's not necessarily impossible for someone with EDS to safely participate in this type of training, but it all depends on the individual. And there can be a high risk of injury and other harm if the exercise isn't right for you or you're not careful. I strongly recommend consulting with an informed medical or movement specialist before proceeding. I just as strongly recommend rejecting the guidance of anyone who doesn't know you and your body but fancies themselves some kind of expert because they have a background in fitness and maybe heard of EDS once. I'd also suggest checking in with EDS community spaces for tips and the support of people who get it.

Speaking from personal experience, I recommend that people who have a tendency to beat themselves up when things aren't going perfectly approach this kind of training with caution when they're in a mood. Safe and effective stretching requires an awareness and acceptance of your limitations and boundaries. If you don't feel like you deserve awareness and acceptance, you might push too hard and too far and end up hurting yourself. Basically, if you get into a position and find yourself thinking something along the lines of "this probably just hurts because I'm doing it wrong, I should just suck it up and suffer," it might be time for you to back off. If you really want to keep going, you could always sulk in child's pose for a while. But you could also substitute your flexibility workout with a head-clearing walk, or rest.

Finally, if you really hate stretching to the point that the thought of it is already making you tune out and shut down, then you don't *have* to do it. You're not unequivocally dooming yourself to a life of poor exercise outcomes and injury if you don't stretch. (Warm-ups and cooldowns do play an important role in performance and injury prevention, but they don't have to include anything that resembles stretching.)

BUST THIS MYTH:
"TOUCH YOUR TOES"

Once upon a time, we treated the distance between a person's upper and lower extremities like it held all the answers to the flexibility. In gyms and schools, we took the sit-and-reach test, in which you sit on the floor, straighten your legs, hinge your hips forward, and measure how far you can reach. In more casual settings, we tried to touch our toes.

The theory was that this measurement could assess how flexible your hamstrings and lumbar spine are. That's not incorrect, but we're now learning that it's incomplete. There are factors besides back and leg mobility, many of them out of your control, that are also in the mix. The length of your limbs might prevent you from being able to reach far enough no matter how flexible you get. The structure of your pelvis and how your hips hinge can also be an issue.

Some fitness experts still use the sit-and-reach and toe touching as general measures of flexibility; if someone can touch their toes, you think "hey, that person has something going right for them in the mobility department." (Unless they're hypermobile and have other things to worry about, but that's a different story.) But there's no need to beat yourself up if that goal is beyond your reach—even if the reason *is* tight hammies or a cranky back. It's not a precise measurement of your flexibility, general fitness level, or worth as a human being.

STRETCHING YOUR UNDERSTANDING OF STRETCHING

The majority of what I've been discussing until this point has been static stretching. As far as I can tell, this method is still the first thing that comes to mind when the average person thinks of stretching. It's definitely what detractors are focusing on when they say that stretching doesn't work. And I do believe it's a great launch pad for a lot of what we're trying to do here. So I figured I'd lead with that.

But there's more to modern flexibility training than the old sit-and-reach. There are different ways to stretch, different ways to think about flexibility and mobility, and different ways to pursue all of the above. Let's start gently sinking deeper into this world (sorry) with a brief overview of some of the most popular types of stretching, what they do, how they feel, and who they might be good for.

The above warnings apply to all of these methods.

STATIC STRETCHING

With static stretching, you move your body into a position that takes a muscle or a group of muscles to the point where you start to feel tension and you hold it for a period of time. Static stretches can be as long or as short as you want them to be, but most experts recommend holding them for somewhere between 20 and 40 seconds. The old-school theory was that holding these positions without moving would overcome the stretch reflex (which regulates muscle length) and allow you to increase the range of your stretches. The new idea is that this time allows your senses to adapt to what's happening—it doesn't change the muscle's capabilities, but it changes how it feels to challenge them. Regardless of the scientific explanation of what's happening, what you do and how that feels remain the same: you move into position, hold, and breathe, and at some point the tension or mild discomfort you're feeling will likely ease a bit. At that point, you have the option to carefully push a little farther, hold again, and keep breathing until it's time to gently release the hold.

For our purposes, the number-one benefit of static stretching is the physical and mental relief that it provides. It can alleviate a little bit of the oppressive heaviness that depression unleashes on your body and take the edge off the tension that anxiety cranks to eleven. It's also a relatively low-effort affair, which makes it a useful tool for those days when you have nothing in the tank but really need a win or a sense that you did *something* with your day.

ASSISTED STRETCHING

There are a couple of different things this term could mean depending on who's using it. If the source is a fitness professional, physical therapist, or exercise nerd, they're most likely using it as an umbrella term for stretching methods that involve contracting and releasing your muscles against an outside force. Proprioceptive neuromuscular facilitation, sometimes called PNF stretching, is the best-known example of this approach. The specifics of PNF will vary with each protocol, but the gist is that another person (like a coach, training partner, or attentive civilian who has been roped into this process for some reason) moves your limb into a stretch and holds it there. You push against the person to contract your muscles at a percentage of your maximum effort for a number of seconds. Then you relax your muscles and the person gently eases your limb further, and you repeat the process.

When I was a new trainer, I was taught that this process overloaded the Golgi tendon organ (the thing that regulates the tension in your muscles) and facilitated a greater range of motion in your flexibility training. But that theory is evolving along with our current understanding of stretching. Some experts believe that PNF stretching could have a greater influence on stretch tolerance than other methods, but all I can tell you for sure is that our ideas about how all this works are in flux.

Outside of PT, I don't think there's much this approach offers the general public that you can't get from other forms of stretching. It's not something you need to worry about unless you like the way it feels or you find it motivational to go down research rabbit holes and geek out about exercise methods. Or unless navigating the awkwardness of the PNF hamstring stretch (it looks . . . a little horny) gives you a temporary mood boost.

More broadly, though, assisted stretching can refer to static stretches that employ outside help. You use a person, a piece of exercise equipment like yoga straps, or a random household item (think belts, towels, or shirts) to help you get into position and stay there. This is something I wholeheartedly recommend.

I don't suggest wrapping a towel around your foot and yanking your leg around in wild abandon. But if you can't get into, hold, or feel remotely comfortable in a position, take whatever props you need to make it work for you. Your body isn't wrong or broken if you need the help and you're not cheating if you use it.

My hamstrings are often tight. Attempting an unassisted supine stretch on them rarely ends well. I lie down, I extend my one leg toward the ceiling, I reach for my calf or thigh, I pull it toward me, and . . . my hands slip. Or I inadvertently shift out of position. Or my knee goes rogue and hyperextends. Or something starts cramping. I get stressed, my upper body starts tensing up, and I descend into a shame spiral. But if I place the middle of a flexband on the sole of my foot, hold the ends in my hands, and gently pull my leg toward me, I get a hamstring stretch that doesn't cause more tension than it eases or trigger an existential crisis.

STATIC AND DYNAMIC STRETCHES

It's always a good idea to watch videos or demonstrations of these moves to make sure you're doing them correctly and to find stretch variations that will achieve the same goals. But to get you started, this list offers a basic full-body set of static stretches and one of dynamic stretches. (I've labeled them by the action involved in the stretch instead of the name to help you focus on what you're doing when you perform these stretches. Anything you do that involves these movements can be a stretch!)

STATIC STRETCHES

- **Open your chest:** With your arms straight out to the sides, draw your shoulder blades together and look up.
- **Round your back:** On hands and knees, let your head drop and draw your spine toward the ceiling.
- **Extend your hips:** While standing straight, kick your left foot toward your behind and grasp it with your left hand. Pull your foot toward your rear. (For a little extra stretch, you can also gently shift your pubic bone forward while staying in this position.) Switch legs.
- **Bend your hips:** While standing, gently bend your right leg and place your left heel on a low table, chair, or step in front of you. Without rounding your back, lean forward and shift your hips back until you feel a stretch through the back of your left leg. Switch sides.

DYNAMIC STRETCHES

- **Circle or swing from the hip sockets:** Swing one leg at a time out, up, or around.
- **Bend at the hip:** Lift your knees to hip height while marching or jogging in place.
- **Straighten at the hip:** Kick your butt while marching or jogging in place.
- **Circle or swing from the shoulders:** Make large or small arm circles.
- **Rotate your spine:** Twist from side to side.
- **Roll your spine down (and stack it up again):** Just like in every yoga and Pilates class.

DYNAMIC STRETCHING

This is a form of active stretching in which you move your body through its full range of motion. (Range of motion, or ROM, means as far as you can go without pain or major discomfort. Not as far as you can go, period. If you're doing moves for your hip sockets, for instance, your ROM will be as far as you can rotate, lift, or swing your leg without pain, discomfort, or clicking/clunking.) Think torso twists, plank walkouts, heel kicks, etc. Basically, if a move involves swinging, rotation, or bending and straightening and you can perform it smoothly with control, you can use it for this method.

Dynamic stretching is especially good at increasing blood flow, literally warming up your muscles, and developing or reinforcing body awareness. This makes it a popular choice for warm-ups, but it has useful applications for mental-health-related issues, too. I find the circulation benefits handy when depression makes me sluggish and zoned out. A brief series of moves is a relatively low-effort thing that I can do to wake myself up a bit. It's not the stretching equivalent of shotgunning an energy drink, but it might make you feel a little more alive.

The body-awareness boost is invaluable if you're trying to build a better relationship with exercise and your body. Putting all your major joints through their ranges of motion is a great way to learn what your parts do and what they feel like when they're doing it without the added pressure of more intense exercise—and any performance anxiety that might come with it. For an example of how that works, try it now with your shoulders. Do a couple of circles forward and then backward at a steady, moderate pace and pay attention to what is happening in your shoulder joints. Now try it again and see if you can focus on how your shoulder blades move to accommodate the action. Can you feel how your muscles work together to move different parts of your body? (If you don't notice anything immediately, please don't stress about it! Developing body awareness is a process. You'll get there.) Admittedly, your level of excitement about this operation will depend on your level of nerdiness. But I went from being a person who was repulsed by fitness and had no awareness or curiosity about the flesh and bones that imprisoned my weary soul to someone who is fascinated by this stuff. I believe it can happen to others, too.

BALLISTIC STRETCHING

Dynamic stretching is sometimes mixed up with another method called ballistic stretching, and some fitness resources list ballistic stretching as a subtype of dynamic stretching. The confusion and conflation come from the fact that both approaches are forms of active stretching that involve moving through your body's ranges of motion. Where they diverge is that dynamic stretching encourages smooth and controlled movements and ballistic stretches involve a lot of fast pulsing, oscillating, and rebounding, which can be incredibly difficult to control unless you really know what you're doing.

Ballistic stretching was big during the high-impact-aerobics era of the 1980s. If you've ever seen the infamous jerky undulations from the original Jane Fonda videotapes, or someone rapidly bouncing up and down while trying to touch their toes, that's what was going on there. But its general popularity faded as most experts concluded that all that bouncing on the joints was doing more harm than good for the average person. It's currently only recommended and used for sports-specific training for elite athletes. As someone who keeps a general eye on fitness trends and philosophies, though, I suspect that ballistic stretching could be on the verge of a comeback, so I wanted to address it here.

If you're reading this in the future and ballistic stretching has been proven to be safe and provide incredible benefits that no other approach to stretching can produce, then by all means go to town. (If you're not a subscriber to *Exercise Trends Monthly*, you'll know this has happened when none of your friends will shut up about the hip new BouncyKnees workout.) If the current position on its risks versus rewards is any more ambiguous than that, here are some things to consider: these moves are challenging to perform well in general, and they become exponentially harder when you're distracted, tired, struggling to be gentle with yourself, working with atypical body awareness, or in a mood. And I've never seen ballistic stretching have physical or mental benefits outside of specialized training that are worth the potential downsides. If there's a workout you'd like to try that has a ballistic component, I suggest skipping the pulses and modifying the stretches into static and dynamic work. That's what I do with the Fondas.

SELF-MYOFASCIAL RELEASE

Translated into everyday words, *self-myofascial release* (SMR) means that you use tools like foam rollers and balls to gently release trigger points and other tight spots in the connective tissue that runs through your body, a.k.a. fascia.

The details vary by method and instructor, but in very general terms you place your weapon of choice on one end of a muscle or group of muscles, lean a moderate amount of your weight into it, and drag yourself across it until you hit a particularly uncomfortable spot. Then you pause, breathe, suffer, curse deities you may or may not believe in, and breathe more until you feel the tension start to ease a little. Then you start rolling again until you hit the next spot.

This might not look like any other kind of stretching, and it'll probably feel different, too. But it's considered part of the stretching family because it's meant to reduce tension and facilitate circulation, flexibility, and mobility.

Foam rolling feels good and provides relief for pain and tension. Or at least it feels good once you hit the relief part; prior to that, it often feels very bad. Given the discomfort-to-comfort ratio involved here, I don't recommend attempting it when you're inclined to push or punish yourself too harshly. But it's a useful exercise for anyone interested in maintaining or improving their general mobility or who desperately needs help relaxing.

If you're willing to get a little geeky about building a better relationship with your body, SMR is a great way to start feeling how interconnected everything inside of us is. I understood how the body worked on a logical level from my training education, but it wasn't until I started rolling one part of my body and felt how that changed other things that I started to *get* it. And if you're willing to get a little earnest about your general mood, you can also use this technique to remind yourself that suffering isn't always permanent. Sometimes things do let up a bit.

A FLEXIBLE ROUTINE

The former trainer in me recommends using static stretching, dynamic stretching, assisted stretching, and SMR to build an effective and satisfying flexibility routine. A well-rounded flexibility program that combines all these methods actually does have the potential to do most of the things that we used to think static stretching accomplished on its own (though not the muscle-lengthening part). The depressed exerciser and reluctant stretcher in me wants to add that you can skip any component that you dislike to the point where you'd rather skip the whole routine than do that component—or where the stress of anticipating or experiencing suffering might undo the relief you'd get from the exercise.

In general, it's wise to do your dynamic work before static and assisted stuff. This will warm up and relax your body and focus your mind, all of which will make setting up and holding your stretches safer and more effective. If you want to include SMR in the proceedings, you can stick it at either the beginning or the end. The foam-rolling faithful tend to believe it should be the first thing you do, because it warms up your tissue and can ease any trouble spots. This is physically true and worth trying if you genuinely love the act of rolling. If you have a love/hate relationship with it, or even a begrudging tolerance, you might be happier wrapping up with it. I know that I don't feel like doing anything after I've rolled.

You can do a workout that's purely dedicated to flexibility and mobility, or you can bookend another workout with your flexibility exercises. Start with dynamic stretching. You can do a general full-body routine, or tailor your stretches to movement patterns that you'll be using in what comes next, like doing arm circles before swimming or doing leg circles and high-knee jogging before kickboxing.

The scientific evidence might not be conclusive on whether a dynamic warm-up has any physical benefits over a cardio one, but anecdotally I find it far more useful for getting your head in the game. Especially when your head is otherwise suffering, obsessing, spiraling, or lightly dissociating. (If you're heavily dissociating, please remember you don't *have* to exercise.) In addition to getting you physically warm and getting your juices flowing, dynamic stretching can wake you up a little and help you (re)connect with your body before you get into more physically and mentally demanding work. If you struggle with changes for any reason, a workout or sports-specific routine can also ease your transition from low activity or inactivity into exercise mode and get you ready for the kind of stuff you'll be doing with your body for the next while. And if you can't get your mind and body going, you can also stop there, because you've still done some stretching and that's great.

Static stretching, on the other hand, is good for cooldowns. It allows you to gently calm your mind and body and smoothly transition from higher-intensity work to a resting state. It's also a useful tool for assessing how you feel as you wind down your workout. If anything feels tense or off during your stretching, make a note of it and keep an eye on it in your future workouts and daily life. If not, just breathe into those stretches and enjoy the release. Optional foam rolling can be added to either end of your routine.

Of course, having a dedicated stretch routine or a dedicated stretch component of your workouts isn't the only way to incorporate flexibility and mobility training into your life. In fact, this type of exercise is particularly well suited to being randomly inserted into your day.

Dynamic stretching can give you a tiny pick-me-up when you're listless and help you shake off some excess energy if you're getting antsy. So many of the moves are easy to do in little pieces while you're doing other things—or when you can't bring yourself to do other things. And you don't have to worry about doing a warm-up first, because stretching can also be your warm-up. Alternate between high-knee marches and heel kicks while wandering around your home. Stand and do a few arm circles and scissors while watching TV—or do them sitting down if you have enough clearance. If you're feeling particularly exasperated and flail-y, twisting your torso to swing your arms from side to side is both a way to rotate your spine and a way to express yourself. If you'd rather not get out of bed, you can turn your nothing-matters-anyway thrashing into dynamic stretches by lying on your back, scooting your feet toward your bum, and shifting your knees from side to side. Or do bed angels— they're like snow angels, but in bed!

There are a number of static stretches that you can do for a sense of accomplishment and degree of relief when you're resting or can't (or don't wanna) do higher levels of activity. Get into child's pose in bed and sigh about the state of the world or your life for a while. On your way out of the bathroom, grab the sides of the doorway with your hands, hold on, and step forward until you feel a stretch in your chest. If you're at a computer, sit up straight, place your right hand on your head and slide your left under your butt (this will function like an anchor and keep your left shoulder from drifting during the stretch). Keep looking at your screen while you pull your head to the right to take some tension out of your neck. Repeat on the other side. (The proliferation of desk-stretch graphics might be a symptom of the nightmares of capitalism and office culture, but the moves themselves are good.) Read a book in downward dog for a while. Or sit cross-legged to open your hips a little. I once took a yoga-for-runners seminar from an instructor who said that her most flexible clients were kindergarten teachers.

Foam rolling can be randomly inserted into your day if you're into that, too. Try keeping a roller close to your desk, sofa, or bed to make it easy to do SMR during downtime.

FLEXIBILITY AND MOBILITY TRAINING

Beyond purely stretching-based workouts, there are also types of exercise that incorporate a strong focus on flexibility and ease of movement into their greater methods. They all have their own philosophies and moves, but they share some important ground: one, they include elements of static holds, dynamic movements, and bodyweight training to develop a balance between mobility and stability in your joints; and two, they're a welcome alternative for anyone who wants to work on their flexibility in theory but can never manage to make themselves stretch.

Here's a quick rundown of your best and most accessible options.

ANIMAL WALKS

Remember doing crab walks as a kid? Some fitness geeks never stopped. And they added a bunch more animal-influenced movements to their arsenal. Put your hands on the floor and run around on all fours like a bear. Squat-jump across the room like a frog. Bend until you touch the ground and walk your hands forward until you're in a plank position. Then scoot your feet toward your hands like an inchworm.

Animal walks have gained traction in children's exercise programs for obvious reasons, but they're catching on with big kids, too. Trainers and instructors embrace them because they're a fun source of functional fitness and because they're a great way to keep group classes challenged and engaged when you don't have a lot of equipment. They can also be adapted for almost any ranges of motion, fitness level, or other needs. Martial artists have adopted them into their warm-ups and cross-training. They're especially popular among grapplers, because their disciplines are all about moving around on the ground in different ways. (By this logic, I think animal movements are also good for people who spend a lot of time flailing on the floor in fits of despair. If you're there anyway, why not try crawling around for a while? If anyone asks you what you're doing, you can say it's sport-specific training.)

As far as brain stuff goes, the biggest asset of animal walking is its playfulness. You're pretending to be an animal! The physical benefits are legit, but the moves themselves are a little silly. It would require a fantastic amount of effort to take the work or yourself too seriously while you're doing them. So you can goof around a little and remind yourself that exercise doesn't always have to be somber and serious. Moving your body can be fun.

Animal walks on their own offer a solid balance of strength and flexibility, but if you're looking for even more focus on the latter, you can also look into animal-movement-inspired workout programs such as Animal Flow and Ginástica Natural, which include yoga and other mobility training influences.

PILATES

Pilates is that core-oriented stuff you do on mats, with small equipment, or on apparatuses that look cool but also kind of torture device-y. This mind-body exercise was developed by gymnast/boxer/bodybuilder/self-defense instructor/circus performer Joseph Pilates in the early twentieth century. Most of his early clients were either dancers or physical therapy and physical rehab patients, and you can see influences of both in current takes on his method. Some modern schools lean more toward the dance aspect, while others go deeper into movement science and physical therapy, so the details might vary among approaches. But the general idea and goals remain the same: use fluid and methodical movements, breathing, and muscle control to develop a balance of mobility and stability. To give you a non-nerdspeak example, in Pilates you want to make the biggest arm circles you possibly can, but you also want to make sure the muscles surrounding your shoulder joint are strong enough to prevent you from ripping your arm of its socket in the process. And you'll probably do something with your core while all of that's happening.

Pilates is the most cue- and instruction-heavy type of exercise I've encountered. It requires a fair amount of body awareness to execute effectively, but the moves and their explanations also help build body awareness. This provides a unique set of benefits and challenges for neurodivergent people and anyone feeling disconnected from their body. Whether or not the balance of the two will be in your favor depends upon your individual needs.

If you think in patterns or find comfort in routines, the way that Pilates moves are sequenced will serve you well. If you need variety to keep yourself stimulated and engaged, it might not be your best option unless you can find an instructor who switches things up frequently. If having something to apply your mind to helps you to shut out intrusive or spiraling thoughts, the level of explanation involved in Pilates can be quite useful. On the other hand, if you have issues focusing, the level of attention required to follow those instructions could wind up frustrating you more than helping you. And if you'd prefer to zone out during your workouts, you'll either be annoyed during a session or unfulfilled at the end of it. There are other exercises that can give you more physical benefits for less constant mental engagement.

Some Pilates concepts can get a little abstract (like when you're prompted to visualize your pelvic floor and then engage it in a way you can't feel, because if you feel it, you're contracting too hard). Most instructors use a lot of metaphors and flowery language to help their students understand what's going on and what it's supposed to feel like. A fantastic amount of thought and experience has gone into these word choices. During my mat Pilates instructor training, one of our teachers went on a fifteen-minute digression about the best way to encourage people to engage their abs when they're lying on their stomach. In her experience, telling people to imagine that there was a fire under their belly button made them flinch and squeeze too hard. When she changed it to picturing an ice cube, they pulled away more gently and achieved the desired amount of tension. These linguistic choices are effective for many populations. For anyone who's been unable to connect with their body through technical language, it can be a useful bridge. The cues can be confounding if you're a more literal thinker, though. They can also be a bit much if you're just not into all that verbiage.

If any of the above sounds like a potential stumbling block for you, that doesn't mean that you can't do Pilates. Maybe it means you don't *want* to, or that you'll be happier considering other mobility exercises. But if you really want to do Pilates, there might be other options out there to help you learn. If following an instructor's cues in classes or videos are a problem for you, a book—or even an instructor's manual—can help you figure out what's going on and how to make that happen in your body at your pace. If regular Pilates classes aren't making sense, an athletic conditioning class designed to help athletes who are used to bigger movement patterns adapt to Pilates moves might be the thing you need.

YOGA

You know, that thing people keep asking you if you've tried.

I'm as tired of the question as you probably are, so I'll spare you the hard sell here. But I think a quick overview is worthwhile. A lot of flagrant yoga recommenders don't seem to understand the practice any better than they understand the life of the person they're recommending it to. (As far as I can tell, they think it's a magic cure for any mental health issue, disability, or chronic illness that makes them feel uncomfortable.) So while you've almost certainly heard that you should try it enough for a few lifetimes, you might be less familiar with what it can actually do, who it can possibly help, and what you might want to consider if it hasn't clicked for you in the past.

Yoga will not fix everything that ails you, but it has the potential to do several good things for your body and brain. Physically, yoga can improve your flexibility, strength, balance, posture, and body awareness. Pranayama, sometimes referred to as "yogic breathing," might contribute to better cardiovascular function. Research into yoga's effect on mood and overall well-being has found that it can have a positive impact on sleep, anger management, stress, self-esteem, cognitive function, PTSD symptoms, and burnout.

Anxiety's also on the list, but I want to add a personal note on that one, as someone who has it—and someone who's discussed the topic with a lot of my fellow anxious people. It's true that a yoga practice can ease some anxiety symptoms, but there's a risk that guided meditation could exacerbate them if you have any issues with focus or perfectionism. If your brain is wired that way, trying to slow it down and follow the instructor's cues can be a challenge. And if it doesn't go well, you can easily spiral from "OK, I'm going to picture this field now . . ." to "Why can't I picture this field?! I bet everyone has a beautiful field in their heads and all I'm doing is thinking even more about not turning my mind off and I'm such a failure and I can't even do this right. How hard is it to picture a field?"

I know guided meditation works wonders for a lot of people. I've seen the serene expressions on their faces when I've snuck peeks at my classmates, desperately trying to figure out if anyone else is struggling. But it's definitely more challenging for some minds than others. What I recommend—and what I am still learning to do myself—is trying to accept that your brain is going to wander more than the instructions recommend. The way I see it, wandering is the closest thing my brain does to rest, and being able to embrace that and not descend into panic is pretty damned meditative.

There's nothing on the list of yoga benefits that you can't get from another type of fitness. You're probably not going to find the same level of meditation that some types of yoga offer, but workouts exist that include visualization exercises, or you can meditate separately from your exercise routine. You won't miss out entirely on something good if you really can't deal with yoga. But yoga does offer an impressive mix of benefits for a single exercise method, so it's well worth trying (or trying again) if you're intrigued. This wide range of benefits is also great news if you happen to love the discipline, but if you're already Team Yoga you probably don't need convincing.

Yoga's wide array of styles—and even wider array of instructors who provide their own interpretations of those styles—also means that there's a very good possibility you'll be able to find a school, instructor, class, video, book, or social media resource that is in line with your beliefs and needs. (There's some evidence to suggest that hatha yoga could be better than other styles for mental health, but it's not so definitive that I'd recommend pursuing it over something else that appeals to you more.) There are options for almost any physical goal and for plenty of mental ones. There are instructors for almost every style, philosophy, and general vibe. There are also an increasing number of amazing options for people who love the idea of yoga but hate colonialism, appropriation, and fitness spaces overrun by skinny white women.

I hope that there's at least one approach to flexibility and mobility in this chapter that appealed to you, or piqued your curiosity enough to try. But if you can't stomach any of it, that's perfectly fine, too. I'm passionate about this kind of training because it's improved my life both as a trainer and as an exerciser, so I want to believe that it can be for everyone. That's me speaking from enthusiasm, though, not authority. I also believe that David Cronenberg films should be for everyone, and practically I know that's not true.

Mobility is important. Being able to move all the different parts of your body with relative ease and lack of pain can reduce injuries and boost your physical and mental health. But workouts with a specific focus on mobility aren't the only way to maintain and improve it. Anything that consistently moves your body in a number of different directions and different ways can do the job. That can be something mentioned above, but it can also be martial arts, dance, gymnastics, or circus training. Or the right combination of exercises from one or both of the next two chapters.

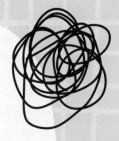

– SIX –

HEAVY STUFF

Carry that weight, as in your
problems but also these weights

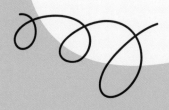

You're already carrying the crushing weight of all your problems. Compared to that, a dumbbell or two is nothing.

Resistance training—a.k.a. strength training, a.k.a. any exercise you perform that makes your muscles contract against an external force, including moves involving free weights, machines, body weight, suspension trainers, resistance bands, isometric holds, medicine balls, and sandbags—can do all sorts of amazing things. I'm assuming that you've heard more than enough about the good it can do for your body. But I've also noticed that most of the resources that discuss the physical benefits of pumping iron go on about weight loss, fat, and calorie burning. So I'm going to provide you with a brief overview that doesn't include any of that nonsense before we get to the good brain stuff you might be less familiar with.

Lifting weights, including your own body weight, makes you stronger. In addition to making you better at picking up heavy stuff—which is pretty cool and useful in and of itself—this can improve your bone and joint health in the present and help to preserve it as you age. Regular weight training can improve your general body mechanics—the way you stand and move in daily life—and might end up boosting your cardiovascular capacity as well. It can also make you look buff, if you're into that and want to pursue it.

In addition, it's starting to look like resistance training can lead to some impressive gains in your mood. Lifting still isn't a cure for mental health issues, but it has the potential to make a much-needed dent in some of them.

Recent studies with a specific focus on the effects of resistance training on mental health have found that lifting can markedly improve depression and anxiety symptoms. (One study found that it can improve symptoms of anxiety in people who don't have an anxiety disorder. So if you're still wondering whether this book applies to you, guess what? There's scientific proof you don't need a diagnosis to benefit from this stuff.)

Perhaps most heartening of all, you don't have to lift a ton to experience these benefits. A 2018 meta-analysis of thirty-three clinical trials concluded that the reduction in depressive symptoms didn't seem to depend on the volume of training or whether the subjects made any measurable strength gains. Performing a basic lifting program twice a week could be enough to get a mood lift too, even if it doesn't give you the glutes of a god.

Experts can't explain how or why this works for sure, but they have some theories. One is that lifting appears to make your brain stronger. In a literal and practical sense, strength training can alter the structure of your brain and how it functions.

The brain isn't a muscle, but as we currently understand it, it kind of responds like one when you start lifting. Resistance training makes your muscles bigger, but it also improves the delivery system that provides muscles with nutrients and strengthens the connections between them and everything else going on in your body. This type of exercise also increases the size of certain parts of the brain, stimulates the development of new blood vessels that deliver nutrients to the brain, cultivates the growth of new brain cells, and strengthens connections throughout your nervous system. And this improvement in how your brain functions could also lead to improvements in how it feels.

Another hypothesis is that resistance training encourages mindfulness. Or maybe it's more accurate to say resistance training *demands* mindfulness. Performing a lift safely and effectively requires you to be present in the moment, especially as those reps grow more tiring and challenging. For some people, the physical sensation of working their muscles in this way can also keep their minds from drifting.

The rush that comes from Doing a Thing probably contributes to lifters' overall sense of well-being, too. The sense of accomplishment you feel at the end of the workout can be an instant mood booster. Seeing your progression over time can make a lasting impact on your self-esteem.

As someone whose depression loves to tell me that nothing I try will ever amount to anything, that last point is huge for me. Strength training has a lot of methodical approaches and a lot of opportunities for linear progression. This means I know I'll be able to see a direct relationship between what I'm putting into it and what I'm getting out of it. It doesn't have to be big things like a personal best or six pack, either. I've enjoyed the flashier moments when they've happened, but it's the smaller, progressive gains that sustain me. If my current progress is stalled, I can also look at the bigger picture, remember how much I could lift when I started, and think of how far I've come.

And if you're not into big-picture stuff, flexing in the mirror and seeing your muscles do their thing is always good for a quick mood-enhancing rush.

WHO SHOULD USE CAUTION WHEN LIFTING?

As a former trainer and someone who continues to harbor strong feelings about weight-lifting technique, my instinctive response is that everyone should be extremely tuned into their bodies when doing this type of exercise. (For more on how to tell when you need to take a rest, see Chapter 8.) There is no good approach to resistance training that requires a person to lift more weight or more times than they're physically comfortable doing. Whether you're training for power, strength, or endurance, the goal is to work responsibly within your ability to gradually change your limits, not to push past them every time you train. Not lifting too much is a fundamental part of the discipline. And if you need more convincing, know that overtraining can also make you sick, hurt you, undermine your gains, and mess with your head.

But as someone who started training when far too many people believed that lifting heavier weights could make women "bulky" and that this was somehow a bad thing, I'll note that you do *not* have to worry about lifting "too much" from an aesthetic or body-image perspective. A lot has changed since I picked up my first dumbbells. Women have broken all sorts of stereotypes and taboos about what we can look like and what we can lift. Trainers and fitness influencers of all genders are doing incredible work to make fitness a place where all body types and all kinds of strength can be celebrated. We now know that building big muscles, for better or worse, just isn't going to happen by surprise. I wish it were that easy, but it's not. For almost everyone, getting really big or really cut requires a lot of specific, dedicated training and eating. (That said, I recommend finding external sources of support and wisdom when beginning a resistance training program if you have any kind of dysphoria or body dysmorphia.)

If, instead, the question is "Which people might want to consider other training options?" the answer is more nuanced. Resistance training isn't considered an outright no-no for any group of people, but there are some who should proceed with caution. Some resources that I've read on Ehlers-Danlos syndrome and hypermobility spectrum disorders recommend a very careful strength training program that uses body weight and equipment other than machines, because that approach is good for strengthening the smaller muscles that stabilize your joints. Others believe that the risk of placing too much stress on your joints and possibly hyperextending them under pressure isn't worth the potential reward. In the end, I think the right answer depends on the individual, their needs and understanding of their own body, and their doctor's recommendations.

And as always, if you're sick or injured or have a condition that you're concerned about, it's wise to consult with a health professional before beginning a new training program.

HOW MUCH, HOW MANY, HOW OFTEN

Picking a strength training goal and calculating out how much you should be lifting, how many times you should lift it, and how often you should repeat it can be incredibly fascinating and motivating if you're into reading up on weight-lifting methods, following tables, and crunching numbers. It can be excruciatingly tedious if you're not.

Based on my experiences at both ends of the muscle-nerd-tolerance spectrum, I believe the best approach here is to give you a general overview. You can use this as a launching pad if you want to go deeper. But if the very thought of doing research for your workout bores you to tears, there's enough in this chapter to guide you through a perfectly functional and useful workout plan. You don't have to think about anything nerdier than that ever again.

If you were my client and I were meeting with you one-on-one, I'd do my best to tailor my explanation and my plans to your personality as well as your goals. Unfortunately, it's not possible for me to do that for everyone who reads these words. But I don't want to suggest a one-size-fits-all approach for everyone. That means you'll have to do a little picking and choosing based on how you like to measure, track, and reward your progress.

The biggest sticking point for most people that I've worked with has been the use of numbers (weight amounts, reps, sets, etc.) in strength training. Some people need them to provide structure and guidance, and some people love them because they're nerds who are into that stuff. Others absolutely cannot abide by the mention of numbers because they find them either discouraging or boring. So while I can't address every single need, I can at least offer guidance for numbers people and for no-numbers people.

If you already know which type you are, please feel free to skip the other answers. Don't even look at them if they're going to make you zone out or put you off strength training! If you don't know your type, read over both and see which approach feels better.

For almost all purposes, there isn't one approach that's better than the other. This is all about finding a way to approach strength training that is going to make you not hate it and maybe even want to do it. However, if you want to get into heavy lifting in particular, I strongly encourage you to go with the numbers, and to save this type of exercise for when you're able to establish and maintain a routine. Being able to consistently work on your strength—and measure progress—will make lifting heavy weights much safer for you. And probably less frustrating, too.

NUMBERS PEOPLE

This part is for math geeks, science nerds, and people who want to know exactly how much they have to do and how far they've come. If you start feeling exhausted just reading this section, skip it and try the no-numbers approach!

How do you figure out how much to lift?

Once you've been lifting for a while, there are mathematical formulas you can use to figure out your one-rep max (literally the most you would be able to lift at one time) and what percentage of that max you'll need to lift to achieve your specific goals. When you're getting started, though, the process is all about trial and error. An experienced trainer might be able to guesstimate where you should start based on observing you and listening to your exercise history and goals, but there's really nothing fancier to the calculation.

What you're looking for is an amount of weight that you'll be able to safely (but not *entirely* comfortably) lift about 10 to 12 times. You want the last couple of reps to feel like a challenge but not a struggle. If you can't finish the set without blowing your form or hurting yourself, you've gone too far. But if getting through those last 2 reps takes a little more concentration and effort and you feel a burn or mild to moderate discomfort, then you're in the right zone. Think of the difference between a grunt or an "ugh" (good) and an "OW!" (too far).

If you have access to multiple levels of weights, whether they come in the form of a machine, a rack of free weights, or a set of adjustable dumbbells, pick an amount of weight that you think you might be able to lift 12 times. Then go down one level: one plate on the machine, one dumbbell size, or one notch on the adjustable dial. The worst that can happen if you lift too light at the start is that you'll get to familiarize yourself with the move—how to do it with good form, and what it generally feels like—without working your muscles to their utmost. The worst that can happen if you go too heavy is that you'll hurt your body and your ego. So start on the light side—you have nothing to prove.

Lift the weight 12 times. If you do end up feeling those last few reps, take a 1-minute rest, and do 2 more sets of 12. If you're not feeling much of anything, rest for a minute and then try again with the next weight up. Repeat as necessary. (If it ends up taking more than 5 sets to find your weight, I suggest calling it a day and continuing the search in your next workout. Sure, it might be a little frustrating when you're ready to get going, but look at it this way: you're stronger than you thought.)

If you don't have access to a wide range of weights, I recommend shifting your focus to how many exercises and how many reps you should be doing instead of how much you should lift. If you're doing bodyweight exercises, for example, you could pick exercises that you enjoy and find a little challenging and figure out how many reps get you into that grunting-but-not-screaming zone, instead of trying to figure out ways to increase weight. If you're lifting a bag of flour or your cat, you figure out how many squats would challenge you instead of trying to source a bigger bag or trading in your kitty for a chonkier model.

How many times do you lift it?

For machine and free weights, 3 sets of 12, with 1 minute of rest between them, is a timeless classic.

There are a lot of different ways to approach reps and sets in weight training, and I encourage you to read up on them and pursue the ones that appeal to you if you're into that. If you're not, or you just want to be told what to do, 3 x 12 is an excellent place to start. Three sets is a fine place to stay, too, if that's what you like. Think of it like ordering a grilled cheese at a diner. There are other things on the menu that are probably great and might be worth trying. But you can't go wrong with the tried-and-true.

For other forms of strength training, you can apply the method in "Break It Up" (see pages 89–94) that works best for you.

How many things do you lift?

There are many answers to this question and I encourage you to explore different training programs and read up on the reasoning behind them if you're into that. If you're not, I recommend a basic full-body workout that includes 1 chest, 1–2 back, 1 shoulder, 1 quads/glutes, and 1 hamstrings/glutes exercise. And if that's still too much thinking about body parts and your flesh prison for your liking, aim for 1–2 pushing-based exercises and 1–2 pulling ones for your upper body, plus 1 move for the front of your legs and 1 for the back of your legs and butt.

How often do you lift it?

You've got a bunch of options here, too. Researching the different ways that you can split up your workout (like leg days and upper-body days, or push routines and pull routines) can be interesting if you get pleasure from thinking about your workouts. It's also useful if you're busy or have scheduling issues and need planning and creativity to fit weights into your life.

If you're not curious and you have no pressing time constraints, though, you can go with twice a week. That's a good frequency for getting started, establishing a routine relatively painlessly, and pursuing those potential brain benefits. You can add a third workout per week if you want to get more serious about the muscular benefits of weight training, too. But remember, these are ideal recommendations for specific goals. If you can only do 1 workout a week—or even half a workout—that's infinitely better than nothing. And you'll still get the satisfaction and mental rush of doing the amount

BUST THIS MYTH:
TRAIN TO THE POINT OF FAILURE

Failure means something very different in strength training than it does in our daily lives.

When I started lifting and people told me to train to the point of failure or fatigue, I assumed that I was supposed to keep lifting until I literally could not move the weights anymore. That was what I tried to do until I started studying to become a personal trainer and one my instructors suggested a different take. Failure, she explained, is when you can no longer continue the exercise *safely and with proper form*.

Say you're doing shoulder presses and you realize that you're starting to compensate by arching your back to get those weights above your head, or you can't control them on the way down again. That's when you're done. You don't keep going until you throw out your back or you drop a weight and it rips your arm out of its socket in the process.

What's more, there are plenty of muscle nerds who don't believe that regularly pushing yourself to failure is a good thing anyway. In their opinion, it can be useful for testing your limits when done sparingly. But it's not going to lead to the same meaningful gains that methodically and responsibly working within those limits does.

Maybe there's a life lesson in that.

you're able to do.

Whatever route you end up taking, try to give the muscles you work during your session at least 48 hours to rest and recover before going at them again. This doesn't mean that you can't do anything for 2 days. For example, you can focus on upper body exercises one day and a leg workout the next. You'll feel and progress a lot better if you don't do the same thing any 2 days in a row. We'll get more into the philosophy behind that warning at the end of this chapter.

What do you do next?

The above is all you'll need to get going. But if you stick with your program long enough, you will be rewarded for your efforts and dedication by having yet more stuff to think about. When you lift regularly, the whole process will eventually start to feel easier—and potentially uninspiring. At that point, you'll need to figure out what you want to do to keep your brain engaged and your muscles responsibly challenged.

Once again, you have a bunch of options for how you can approach this. If charts and detailed guidance are your thing, you are going to love learning about how to cycle and periodize your workouts for different goals and how that changes the weight you're lifting, and the reps and sets you're doing. My autistic brain flourished when I was poring over charts, calculating my abilities, and drawing up strength and endurance phases in my training program when I was in my serious-business-lifting phase.

But being serious about lifting takes a lot of mental effort to research, mull over, and execute. If you're not enthralled by the process—or you're not hiring someone else to do it for you—it can easily feel like yet another mind- and soul-draining demand in your miserable life. Even if it's not terrible for you, the planning could be a slog. Or intriguing in the abstract, but way more than you can commit to right now.

Mercifully, there's another way to progressively challenge yourself in strength training that is practical, easy to follow, and doesn't require a lot of planning on your part—or much extra thought at all, for that matter. (It served me well when I was first starting out, and it's working for me now that I'm tentatively rekindling my love affair with lifting.) Start with your 12 reps. When that gets easy, aim for 15 reps. When that no longer poses a challenge for you, move to the next weight up and drop your reps to 8. Then work up to 10. Then back to 12. And so on. (At any point, if one day you simply can't stomach the thought of your regular routine, you can always switch it up and try lifting lighter weights or doing fewer sets, or trying a body-weight work-out for a change. You don't have to be growing, building, and improving every time you lift. You can just be exerting yourself because it gives you a little blip of good brain chemicals.)

NO-NUMBERS PEOPLE

This section's for the ungovernable, the math haters, and everyone else who didn't even want to look at the numbers section. (For some reason this approach gets a bad rap, so let me say for the record that you are just as virtuous and valuable as the number-motivated!)

What kind of strength training should you do?

One of the great things about getting away from hard numbers in your strength training is that it allows you to rethink what can be considered strength training. If you're in a weight room, you'll probably want to stick to more traditional weight-lifting moves. But if you're hanging out in an empty studio, at home, or in a park and just want to Do a Thing, you've got a ton of options. Anything that makes your muscles work can be strength training and can potentially give you that brain rush you're chasing. So you can do push-ups, but you can also bench-press your weighted blanket. You can do squats, or you can sit against a wall with your thighs parallel to the floor to watch TV. You can look up structured routines to do with a medicine ball or you can throw one around for fun.

Feel free to get creative. You have all of traditional weight training, functional training, body-weight training, and general stuff that moves your body at your disposal. Just don't do anything that is unsafe or hurts you.

Ideally, I would suggest that you aim for balance in the moves you choose. If you love doing moves that work your chest, for example, try to also find a move you enjoy (or feel all right about) that works your back. Or balance the work you do on the muscles in the front of your legs with working the ones in your hamstrings and calves. You don't have to do this if you really can't stomach it, to the point that you'd rather give up chest exercises than add a back one. But in general, you'll be more comfortable and safer if you try to balance out your moves.

How much strength training should you do?

When you get away from numbers in strength training, I find it helpful to shift your focus from the exact amount you should be lifting to the amount of exercise that will help you pursue your goals. With this approach, you'll still be aiming to challenge yourself and develop strength and positive brain vibes. But the way you try to get there will be a little different. Instead of doing a group of exercises that involve lifting X pounds Y times for Z sets, you're going to focus on the feeling that you get from each exercise.

The goal here is to find an amount that challenges you without beating you up. In the numbers section, I described this as the difference between a grunt or an "ugh" and an "OW!" The same applies here.

For an example of what that would look and feel like in action, let's say you're doing squats with either the weight of your own body or something you can safely hold while you perform the exercise (such as a bag of flour, a small- or medium-sized medicine ball, or an amenable pet). You'd aim to keep going until your last couple of squats burn and feel a little harder than the previous ones, not to the point where your legs turn to complete jelly and you feel like you're going to collapse. And you definitely want to stop if you notice your form starting to slip. When you can no longer perform the move safely, you're done.

In terms of workout structure, everything we covered in Chapter 4 can still apply here. Pick the style that works best for you and apply your strength training moves to it. Then do an amount that gets you into that challenged-but-not-destroyed zone. And definitely stop if you can't do it safely anymore.

If that's still too much to deal with, you can always take it one move at a time. If doing a whole workout or a whole set is too much to think about, tell yourself that you'll start with a single rep and see how that goes. If it feels tolerable, try another one. And so on.

If that still feels like too much, lie down on the floor and have a brief time-out, snit, or pout, whichever suits your current situation. Then get up. Then lie down again. Repeat if you're so inclined. Because getting up is a strength exercise, too.

How often should you strength train?

I discussed what the studies say about getting mental health benefits from weight lifting in the beginning of this chapter, so I'm not going to make you go over them again here. If the frequency mentioned in those studies (two times a week) feels manageable, that's great. Go with that.

If that feels like too much for you right now, please don't panic. And don't give up. Do what you can when you can. Everything we've covered so far applies here. The amount you can do is a million times better than the amount that makes you never want to start.

What do you do next?

Whatever you want, really. If you're happy doing your strength-training thing, whatever that turns out to be, you can keep doing it forever. Or you can decide to experiment with other exercises and workouts. If you ever find yourself thinking you'd like to try something with more structure, you can revisit the advice for working with numbers. If not, you never have to think about them and can continue to do whatever your mind and body feel up to.

LIFTING AT THE GYM

Gyms are filled with large selections of equipment that you can use for resistance training. They're also populated by other people who are using them for similar purposes and people employed to help all of you use them. This can be a blessing or an enormous curse, depending on how prepared you are to be perceived (or, perhaps even worse, helped) by other people. Here are some tips for navigating the weight-lifting options.

WEIGHT MACHINES

Those big things on the gym floor that are strictly dedicated to 1 or 2 moves each are an excellent place to start if you've never lifted before. They're fairly instinctual to use and most have written instructions and diagrams on them that can help if you're confused about a particular detail. This also makes them a good choice for days when your brain is feeling a little foggy or your body awareness feels a touch off.

If you've ever paid attention to weight training, you've probably heard the argument that weight machines are inferior to free weights. That's not true. There are advantages and disadvantages to both, and it's worth reading up on the pros and cons if you want to pursue specific goals in your training. For general mental well-being and the goals we're talking about in this book, though, the choices are almost equal in terms of benefits, and you don't have to think any further about it if you don't want to.

If you have questions or concerns about the machines while you're at the gym, someone on the gym floor or at the front desk should be able to address them. I appreciate how nerve-racking this prospect might be. I used to be one of those official gym-floor people and I still get anxious at the thought of talking to one (though in fairness, talking to almost anyone makes me anxious). So I won't try to tell you that it's going to be easy. But what I can say for sure is that it is part of their job to help you with those things and you will not look weird or silly if you take them up on it. They would much rather you ask for help than hurt yourself. I can also assure you that they've heard and dealt with issues far weirder and more annoying that anything you could come up with and they will not think you're the worst. (Gym bros who don't put their weights back after using them and force the gym staff to clean up after them are the worst.) And if you really don't want to talk to anyone, you can always look stuff up on your phone.

FREE WEIGHTS

In most gyms, you'll find a chunk of space off to the side of the machine floor that's packed with dumbbells, plates, barbells, benches, and racks. That's the free weight area. ("Free" in this case refers to the fact that the weights aren't attached to other pieces of equipment, not to how much you're paying for the privilege of having access to them.) It's a great place to check out if you're curious about using this equipment and something you ignore if you're not.

As I said above, free weights are almost equal to machines if you're just trying to soothe your brain by breaking a sweat. But free weights might have a slight advantage if you're specifically looking to increase your body awareness. Lifting dumbbells and bars without the support and guidance of a machine will foster a different level of physical and mental understanding about what you're doing in a move and what it feels like, both in the targeted muscles and in the rest of your body. It can be a rewarding experience, but if you do choose this route, I want you to be aware that there can also be quite a learning curve. Free-weight exercises will recruit your core and the smaller muscles that stabilize your joints, and it's going to take some practice to strengthen and coordinate everything. So if you pick up the weights, get set to lift, and then find yourself wondering what the hell is going on, that's normal. It will start to make more sense and feel more natural in time.

If you're learning about free-weight training on your own, in the early days I recommend consulting sources that provide basic information and not a lot of editorializing. Look for instructions that will simply tell you how to do a move and what muscles it works, from sources such as strength-training anatomy books or functional, fact-based websites. Blogs, forums, specialty magazines, and many exercise books are likely to get into discussion of variations, esoteric debates about form, and "perfect" exercises for various body parts, but it will be easier for you to figure out how to safely execute a move and what it feels like in your body without all that extra noise. And digging into all that other stuff will be less overwhelming and intimidating when you've established your own relationship with your body and the basics.

FUNCTIONAL TRAINING

A number of gyms have another area—or a separate studio—that features a collection of cable machines, mats, suspension trainers, balls of both the Swiss and medicine variety, and other random bits of small equipment. This might be called the functional training area. Officially, functional training is a style of resistance training that focuses on movement patterns you make in your daily life, undertaken to help you function better and prevent injuries in those real-life tasks. But sometimes it means "training involving the stuff we didn't know where else to put."

For our purposes, the main benefit of the various things in this area are the variety they can add to your workouts. A couple of moves using the equipment you find there can be a nice change of pace from more traditional strength training. They might even be fun, depending on your mood and your fondness for the greater world of weight lifting. If you are interested in anything you see in that corner, try adding an exercise or two to the end of your workout. (You may really have to ask for help on this one, since cable machines don't often have the same posted instructions as weight machines, and other equipment has even less—but you can also spot something that seems intriguing, look it up yourself at home, and come back next time prepared with moves to try.) If you're not interested, or you just don't feel like mixing it up today, skip the fancy stuff and grab a mat. The other benefit of functional training areas is that they're usually a good location for warm-up and cooldown activities.

TRAINERS

Most commercial gyms—and some community-based YMCA-style ones—will try to sell you personal training packages. And they'll try *hard*. If you're not interested, you're going to have to be prepared to say no. Maybe more than once. The first thing they'll probably do is offer you an orientation or trial session that's included with your membership. I strongly recommend taking that, because it's an important opportunity to get a general sense of your new gym, guidance on how the machines work, and some one-on-one feedback about how you're using them. (If they offer any kind of assessment along with that session, I recommend skipping that part unless you really want to go through being weighed and measured and talking about goals that come with specific numeric measurements. And if they tell you that you can't skip that part, run. That's not a good gym for you.)

You do not have to do a full workout during an orientation session. But in order to familiarize yourself with the equipment and make sure that you're using it safely, you will have to try a few reps and you will have to deal with a trained professional watching you do those reps and offering you suggestions. You might have the option of doing a full workout, but you can also be clear up front if you just want to be shown a few things and make sure you're not hurting yourself while you're doing them. If you're uncomfortable saying that, then I think the stress involved in the situation will outweigh the benefits for you personally, and you can skip it. And if you do feel strong enough to ask for this and the trainer doesn't respect your boundaries, skip the session for sure.

In any event, be aware that there's probably going to be an upsell at the end, and you will need to politely but firmly say that you're not interested.

Practice it beforehand if you need to.

Keep an eye out for trainers who are walking around the gym floor. This is a real job that serves a vital function in fitness establishments. These people are there to offer basic assistance when asked, make sure that everyone is being safe in their movements and respectful to one another, and put away equipment that ignorant gym bros have left lying around after they're done with it. But some gyms will try to sneak covert sales into that list of duties. A small but unfortunate percentage of those places will also coach the trainers to essentially neg you into purchasing their services. So they'll criticize what you're doing to make you believe that you're wasting your time if you don't hire them.

I haven't met a single trainer who loves this part of the job, not even the soft-sell version where they don't have to be mean. Helping people is great. The rest is mortifying and completely outside of what they want to be doing with their expertise and passion. There's a good chance that they'll be more than happy to move on if you simply thank them for their advice. (And if they're not, you're well within your rights to tell them to back off. This may be hard if you don't like confrontation or worry about judgment from Fitness People, but if there's anything a trainer should respect, it's a firm "OK, I need to go back to my workout now.")

That takes care of how you can manage the interactions externally, but I think it's also important to address how you can process them internally. Remember that this is not a commentary on your lack of skill if someone singles you out and that there's no reason to feel ashamed or discouraged. Think of it like salespeople who try to give you cosmetics samples at mall kiosks. They're not doing it because they think your hair and skin are gross. This is more about them trying to convince you that their services are valuable to you than it is about what you're doing. If a trainer offers a tip about safety, then that's worth considering. But if the tips are about gains or anything else, and *especially* if they're attached to a pitch about paying for tips about gains, you can take what's useful to you and chuck the rest.

If you are interested in hiring a trainer, these interactions can become part of your feeling-out process. If you luck out and click with the trainer providing your orientation, or you find a trainer on the floor particularly helpful, you might not have to search further. Find out their availability, and if that works for you, book a single session to start. If that goes well, you can consider making a longer-term commitment and buying a package of sessions.

If these opportunities don't pan out or don't feel quite right, visit the front desk and ask who else is available. It's also worth finding out if your gym allows outside trainers. You might have a chance to cast a wider net in your search and start looking online and asking friends if they can recommend anyone who would be a good fit for you.

Take note of what you didn't like—and what you liked, if there is anything—about the trainers you've met so far and make a list of what you want. Be clear about your goals and your boundaries. This will help gym administrators make the best recommendations for you and be a good litmus test for you. A suitable trainer will welcome this information, because knowing more about you means they'll be better able to tailor a program to your needs. Any trainer who balks at your requests has already proven themselves to be the wrong one for you.

You don't have to be confrontational during your trainer search, but you should be firm and clear about what you want and what you don't. If you are anxious or shy or have problems standing up for yourself, try to schedule your search for times when you don't have a lot of other demands. Or bring someone along to support you. (If they don't belong to the gym, you can ask to have this conversation at the front desk, or see if your gym offers free or discounted guest passes to members.) Practice if you need to. I don't believe that a lot of good comes out of pushing yourself completely out of your comfort zone (the edge of your comfort zone is where the magic happens) but this is an exception. It actually is worth some extra discomfort and extra demands on your mental bandwidth to make sure you're getting what you want.

All of the above can apply to taking classes, too. Try what interests you.

Return to what you like. Move on from what you don't. If you're not sure about a class, you also have the option of asking if you can talk to the instructor before you give it a try.

Of course, just because the above suggestions sound relatively straightforward on paper doesn't mean they're easy to apply to real life. Especially when you're already exhausted, demoralized, or stretched too thin. It's a little like finding the right therapist. The end result can be a net positive for your mental health, but all of the research and effort that goes into the process can take a significant mental toll.

I'm making these suggestions because they're useful for people who either have the energy to put into figuring this stuff out or figure that mustering the energy will eventually be worth it for them. If you're not in one of those categories, that's perfectly fine too. You can put this advice aside and deal with it either when you're feeling up to the task or when it starts to feel worth it. Or never think about it at all, go sign up for a membership, and do your own thing when you can.

GYM BROS (and other unpleasant gym denizens)

There are two types of hyperdedicated fitness people you'll find at the average gym. The first is the muscle nerds. These types are harmless. They might look intimidating, with their big lifts and their bodies that look like they walked straight out of an anatomy textbook. But they got that way because they're extremely dedicated to the activity. Training is something they genuinely love, and a large portion of their lives, including their diets, revolve around it. (I say this with love, but I think that being a dedicated gym person at that level has far more in common with trainspotting or getting deep into baseball stats than it does with other athletic pursuits. It's all about numbers and timing and keeping detailed and minute observations. Our society just treats gym dedication differently because it often results in a body type that our current culture values.) If you ever feel weird around them, just remember that they're probably not thinking about you at all. They're visualizing their next set or counting down the minutes to their next protein shake.

Gym bros (who can be any gender, by the way) are far more annoying. They're the ones who act like they own the place. They leave equipment lying around after they're done with it. They hover intimidatingly near equipment that other people are already using, as if we're supposed to drop what we're doing and cede everything to the more deserving exercisers. They make snide comments about other people at the gym. Or worse, they offer viciously patronizing encouragement.

Unfortunately, I don't have substantial advice for dealing with these dicks. From what I've been able to observe, the problem is getting better. Whether people are getting less assoholic or gyms are getting better about fostering more inclusive and welcoming environments, I don't know. But I have noticed a gradual shift in what I've seen and what other people I know have experienced. These characters haven't gone away entirely, though.

I can tell you that anyone who cares about what someone else is doing or what they look like at a gym is an insecure little baby. And anyone who can't take pride in their own fitness-related accomplishments unless they feel like they're doing something that other people can't or won't is empty inside. But I know that's not enough to completely defang them in the moment.

You're well within your rights to tell them to eff off. If one of them asks to work in (that is, use the machine while you're resting between sets and vice versa), it is good gym etiquette to consider it, but you don't *owe* them that, either. It's also understandable, albeit entirely unfair to you, if you would prefer to work out somewhere else to avoid them.

Whatever you do, don't listen to their exercise advice and don't copy any of their exercises. Very few of them have a clue what the hell they're doing.

LIFTING AT HOME

Your home has no gym bros, which is an unmitigated good. It's also full of opportunities for less-conventional training options that you might not feel comfortable doing at the gym or don't have time to do at the gym. At home, you can do little bits of your workout throughout your day. You can try a rep or two of something and keep going if you get into the groove or move on to something else or stop if it's not clicking. You can have fun lifting household objects. You can do strength training in bed if you want to!

One thing you won't have at home, though, is a huge selection of cool equipment. That's not necessarily bad, but it will take some creative planning to work around if you want to get deeper into strength training.

My suggestions for how much to lift and how to plan and progress your workouts still apply here (see pages 131–138 if you need a refresher). So do my tips about looking for a personal trainer, if you choose to hire a trainer to come into your home (virtually or IRL) and make you do stuff. And everything else we've covered throughout the book about breaking workouts into manageable pieces and doing what you can 1,000 percent still applies here. The only difference is figuring out what you can lift in a home environment, how large a collection of cool equipment you want, and what should go in it.

THE BASICS

Unless you have the budget and want to build a full-blown home gym and dive into a full-blown strength-training program, I recommend starting small. Once you're sure that you like working out at home—or are begrudgingly willing to keep going, anyway—you can start to add to your arsenal. At that point, you can be more certain that you're going to use what you buy and that it will be worth the investment. You'll probably have a better understanding of what kind of resistance exercises are enjoyable and useful for you, which will help you figure out what kind of equipment you want to invest in.

IF IT'S HEAVY, IT'S A WEIGHT

You don't need to buy fancy gear to get the mood-lifting benefits of weight training. Repeatedly lifting anything heavy will get you at least a few good brain chemicals. To go completely equipment free, try one of these exercises.

- **Goblet squat your pet.** Pick up a consenting cat or dog in your arms, stand with your feet shoulder width apart, and slowly bend your knees until your thighs are parallel to the floor. Repeat until your pet wants to be put down.
- **Row your groceries.** With a full bag in each hand, keep your back straight and bend forward from your hips (think of lightly drawing your belly button toward your spine to support your lower back). Keeping your elbows close to your sides, pull your bags up until your biceps are parallel with your torso. Then slowly lower them. Repeat 12 times, or until you're worried the ice cream will melt.
- **Hammer curl your cocktail (or mocktail).** A full 750-milliliter bottle of liquor or juice weighs about 3 pounds. Before you mix up your drink, hold the bottle in one hand with your arm down at your side and lift up and forward, hinging at the elbow. Repeat 12 times per side or until you're thirsty. (It's a common joke among muscle nerds that you do hammer curls to strengthen your drinking muscles.)

- **Bench-press your weighted blanket.** If you're not ready to get out of bed, roll a weighted blanket into a bolster shape. Lying on your back and facing the ceiling, push up the bolster from your chest until your arms are straight, then slowly lower. Repeat whatever amount of times. If you don't want to get out of bed, I'm not going to make you think about numbers or hard minimums.

To start an at-home resistance program, you need only two pieces of equipment: a yoga mat or a set of puzzle-piece mats to stand and roll around on, and something that you can use for pulling-based exercises that will target your upper back.

There are amazing body-weight exercises that will target the rest of your body. These moves are wonderful for cultivating body awareness, waking up all the smaller stabilizing muscles, and building and toning the bigger ones. But unless you're a prodigy who can instantly do pull-ups and you have a random bar in your abode you can use for these purposes, you're going to need gear specifically for your lats, traps, and rhomboids. I suggest one of the following three options:

- **Flexband or tubing:** A.k.a. the big elastics that you use for strength-training purposes. Flexbands are the flat kind and tubing is round with handles. With a little ingenuity, you can use either of these for makeshift lat pull-downs, rows, and reverse flies. They take up next to no space and they're inexpensive. You can get one at your average dollar store these days. (Although as you progress you'll want to graduate to the kind you can get at fitness-supply stores for both strengthening and safety reasons.)

- **Dumbbells:** Weights that are meant to be used one per hand (versus barbells, which are two-handers). With one set of these, you can perform bent-over and one-arm rows just like you would at a gym. Dumbbells get progressively more expensive—and more annoying to store at home—as they get bigger. But a set in the range of 7.5 to 20 pounds range, which is a good starting range for rows, will be reasonably priced. A secondhand set will be even cheaper. And they don't take up much room; you can stash them in a corner.

- **Suspension trainer:** This is the thing made of adjustable nylon straps that you can anchor over a door or hang from a mount on a wall or ceiling. You might also know them as TRX, which is a brand name. They're good for rows, reverse flies, and exercises designed to gradually prepare you for a full pull-up. A suspension trainer costs a bit more than the other two options, but it's still relatively affordable, especially if you look for secondhand or generic options. (You should not make your own unless you really know what you're doing. Don't ask me how I know that.) Both the wall-mount and door-hook options are safe, effective, and painless to set up, take down, and store.

As you progress in your body-weight training, you'll be able to use your equipment choice to challenge other major muscle groups, too. Then you can start thinking about other equipment worth investing in.

GOOD INVESTMENTS

Unless you have a big budget and a bigger home, assembling an entire free-weight section or getting machines is wildly impractical. With the current state of at-home equipment, though, you can approximate a good chunk of what you'd be able to do with that setup with only a few key pieces.

First, consider investing in a piece of equipment that will let you work progressively through multiple exercises. Like a suspension trainer, where changing the angle or position of a move can alter the degree of resistance involved. Or a set of adjustable dumbbells. Or a cable machine designed for home use, if you have the space and really want to splurge.

You can stop there, or you can supplement your workouts with smaller equipment along the lines of what you'd find in the functional training section of a gym. This part comes down to preference and what you think you'd enjoy. Do you want a medicine ball to throw around a local park on warm days or roll around with at home? A pair of stability cushions because you've discovered that you like a good balance challenge? A kettlebell to start swinging? Go for it.

Brand-name models aren't a necessity for any of these products. For durability's sake, I don't recommend getting the cheapest ones on the market. But there's not much that the most expensive options could offer that you wouldn't get from a solid midrange purchase. Also check out used goods online and at thrift stores and fire sales. There is almost always a gym going out of business or an individual getting out of fitness who is looking to unload their equipment for a fraction of the ticket price.

NO PAIN, YES GAIN

Now you know how to start strength training and how to keep going. Before we move on, here are some tips that will help you get the most out of your resistance workouts without taking too much out of you.

- **Rest.** There is zero downside to resting in strength training. Not only does it prevent injuries and keep you from feeling like a complete zombie, it's also what makes gains happen. When you lift a weight, the action makes tiny tears in your muscle fibers. When you rest and refuel, those fibers heal and become bigger and stronger. If you don't rest, your muscles never have a chance to grow.

- **Don't push yourself past your breaking point.** You don't even have to push yourself *to* your breaking point. You should keep lifting only as long as you can lift while maintaining safe and proper form, not until you can't lift at all. Discomfort and a touch of burning is OK. Pain is *not*. All the gains that you'll make in strength training come when you test your capabilities, not your limits.

- **Have a backup plan.** In general, it's wise to have a modification or two in the back of your mind just in case a move isn't going as planned or feels off for any reason. But this is especially important when you have any kind of issues that might mess with your focus during more challenging moves. Sometimes I enjoy doing full ass-to-grass squats (which is what it sounds like—super-deep squatting until your butt almost touches the ground). I've read up on the reasoning and function behind this move, and I like the way they feel when I do them. When I'm feeling aware and sharp, I can execute them well without doing anything to endanger my lower back and knees. If I'm feeling foggy, I notice that my form gets a little sloppier and things start feeling weird. When that happens, I switch to parallel squats (squatting until your thighs are parallel to the floor and then returning to standing), which I have a lot more practice with and are easier for me to control.

- Engage your core. You don't have to contract the hell out of everything and lift like you're wearing a tightly laced flesh corset. But a little activation of your core will help support your back during lifts that put pressure on the core and will keep your form better overall. If you don't know what that should feel like, stand up, exhale, and think of lightly drawing your belly button in the general direction of your spine. That's the level of engagement you're aiming for.

- Try not to tense up. I'm sorry to throw this one at you. I'm a perfectionist with anxiety, so I know the suggestion is only going to add to your potential stress. But I also have a lot of personal experience with this problem, and I know my body feels better when I do find a good balance. Paying attention to form and making sure that everything's working the way it should be is extremely important. But if you start to stress about it, you'll end up carrying a lot of that stress in your shoulders. They'll start creeping upward, and your neck will end up feeling pretty crappy. Don't worry about this too much, because overthinking it will only add to your stress, but if you notice that your shoulders are almost touching your ears, take a moment to relax them and glide them down again.

- Rest. Yes, we discussed this one already, but it's really that important. If you're still not convinced, there's a whole chapter dedicated to it starting on page 175.

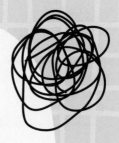

– SEVEN –

RUN FROM YOUR PROBLEMS

Getting your heart rate up
without having an anxiety attack

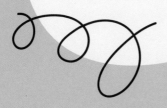

When you hang out with recreational runners, you learn all sorts of weird and interesting things. Like which races have the best swag bags and postrun snacks. And where to poop and what leaves are safe to wipe with when there are no public toilets on your long run route. And everything that can go wrong below the waist when the muscles and connective tissues that keep the knee in place aren't in balance.

You'll also learn that a large percentage of runners have emotional issues. This isn't an insult. They're often the first to admit it, sometimes with impressive levels of self-awareness and acceptance. Many runners are quite open about the therapeutic role that running plays in their lives.

That's right: you can literally run from your problems. The majority of runners I know—myself included—started putting in physical mileage because we were trying to get some figurative distance between our minds and something going on in our lives. None of us have ever outrun our demons, but we have found some clarity and relief in the run itself, at least in retrospect (it's a perfectly normal runner thing to hate running but love *having* run). During better times, we even find some goals to run toward.

But you don't have to become a serious runner to get a mood boost from cardiovascular exercise. Anything that brings your heart rate up and keeps it there for a time can be cardio, with all the brain benefits that entails. Walking to the corner store to get a snack can be cardio. (Walking in general is an amazing form of cardio and deserves so much more respect than it gets.)

One-person dance parties are cardio. Waving your arms above your head while decrying the state of the world or thinking about how much you hate cardio can be cardio, if you do it hard enough and keep it up long enough. Anything that gets and keeps your heart beating a little faster can have a positive impact on your physical and mental well-being.

And it really can be just a little faster. I've noticed that a lot of people seem to assume that all cardio involves gasping for breath while your heart pounds in your chest. Some forms of cardiovascular training include parts where you push yourself to that level (and responsibly bring your heart rate back down again), but you absolutely do not have to push yourself that hard to get a good cardiovascular workout.

If you don't know what making your heart beat a little faster feels like, try this: Find your pulse right now. You don't have to count it, just try to feel the rhythm of it. Now stand up and move a bit, like marching on the spot or taking a small dance break. No burpees. When you're done, find your pulse again and notice the change. That's getting your heart rate up. That's all you need.

Cardiovascular exercise does wonders for the system it's named after. It strengthens the heart, increases lung capacity, and improves blood flow. It can also support better brain function, top up your energy levels, make you sleep better, and aid in illness and injury prevention. All of which can contribute to a better headspace.

Scientifically speaking, studies have found that cardio can reduce symptoms of anxiety, depression, and negative moods. Experts believe it can increase self-esteem and cut down on feelings of isolation or loneliness. And anecdotally, I've noticed other benefits with my clients, my training buddies, and myself.

Steady-state cardio—the low- or medium-intensity stuff that involves a consistent pace and effort level throughout the workout—is especially good for clearing your head. First, it requires you to tune out distractions because you can't safely or effectively move your body in this manner while, say, tinkering on your phone every few seconds (a completely hypothetical example that's not ripped from my doomscrolling-ridden life). Once you've made that separation, there are a few different things you can do with your mind. You can try some light meditation by mindfully focusing on the sights and sounds around you, or repeating a mantra in your head. A string of curses works just as well if you like the idea of working on focus but you struggle with mindfulness exercises. You can also let your mind wander and see where that takes you. And if that doesn't work, you can always look for a more entertaining form of distraction to keep you going, such as music, a podcast, or an audiobook. (See "What to Listen to at the Gym" on page 162 for ideas.)

Group exercise that primarily focuses on steady-state training, such as running groups or dance classes, is a good choice for anyone who longs for the camaraderie that some people get from team sports without the pressure of having other people depend on you to do things well. Group dynamics and competition might be an issue, because they always are when humans assemble, but there's a very good chance that you'll be able to just vibe around each other while pursuing your own cardio goals. As an autistic person, I like to think of these activities as parallel play for adults. If you can stand crowds, participating in races for the sake of doing them, a.k.a. racing to "complete, not compete," can do that for you, too.

Interval training—the stuff that alternates between short bursts of higher-intensity work and longer periods of low- to medium-intensity recovery activity—is great for almost instant distraction and stress relief. A little bit of hard cardio can blow off a lot of steam. Interval training is the most cathartic form of exercise I've ever done. And it's almost impossible for your mind to fixate on negative thoughts when you're too busy reminding yourself to breathe, assuring yourself that the difficult parts don't last forever, and counting down to your next rest. There's also a decent possibility that your brain will be too tired to wind itself up again at the end of your session.

WHO SHOULD USE CAUTION WITH CARDIO?

Once again, I say it's important for everyone to make sure they're not overexerting themselves. I believe this warning is particularly important when it comes to cardio, because people who get into this form of exercise tend to get *really* into it. And I've never come away from talking to a member of the faithful thinking "wow, that person has an unimpeachable sense of proportion."

If you find yourself getting excited about cardio, you will have to strike a balance between indulging your newfound enthusiasm—a genuinely good thing—and preventing yourself from pushing too hard. Adding too much intensity or too much distance too soon will greatly increase your risk of illness or injury, which will make you feel bad and be a real kick in the junk for your motivation.

You'll also want to keep an eye on the number of cardio sessions and the total amount of time and/or mileage you're doing a week. If you push yourself too hard or for too long, you could easily end up undermining the mental health benefits you might be getting from your workouts. Symptoms of overtraining include soreness, strains, chronic overuse injuries, illness, concentration issues, fatigue, irritability, low sex drive, and other complete mood ruiners. (If you're more of a cardio tolerator than a lover, at least you'll probably never have to worry about this.)

If you hang out with Fitness People you may encounter a claim that you shouldn't do too much cardio because it leads to weight gain. If anyone says this, you can ignore them or yell at them for buying into fatphobic myths and not understanding or caring how our bodies really work. "Cardio makes you fat" is like "vaccines give you autism." They don't, but there's absolutely nothing wrong with being those things, anyway.

As great as cardio can be for anxiety, it does come with one possible complication. That rising heart rate and the body's responses to it might be a little too close to what happens in an anxiety attack for everyone's liking. They can even trigger attacks in some people. The benefits vastly outweigh the risks, and I don't want anyone to avoid any type of movement that gets your heart rate up. (Personally, I find it helpful to do cardio when I'm feeling panicky, because it means my higher heart rate feels explicable and in my control.) But I do recommend starting slowly and noting how it makes your brain and body feel. You don't need to be hypervigilant, because that's only going to make you more anxious. But a general awareness is a good idea. If cardio exercise does exacerbate your anxiety, it's entirely up to you whether you want to try to work through it or look for an alternative that doesn't require the extra stress and work. They're equally valid options. And whatever you choose, please be gentle with yourself.

And again, if you're sick, injured, or have another condition that you're concerned about, it's wise to consult with a health professional before beginning a new training program.

CARDIO AT THE GYM

When you walk into the average gym, you will see a bank of cardio machines. There will be plenty of treadmills and elliptical trainers, and perhaps a small herd of stationary and recumbent bikes. Often you'll find a random piece of less familiar equipment lurking in a corner somewhere. Any of these machines will get your heart rate up and enable you to pursue all the mental health benefits of cardio training. Some might be better choices than others for specific physical or mental needs (or simply more to your personal taste), so there's a few general tips to keep in mind when you're looking for the right machine for you.

Treadmills are easy and practical to use. If you don't want to get into any fancy features or programs, you can step on, put on the safety clip (I don't care if it makes you feel silly, it's for your own good; if you slip, which is unlikely but possible, that tiny safety measure will stop the treadmill and save you from flying off the back, hurting yourself, and becoming the star of a viral video), press start, and then gradually up the speed until you find your zone. If you're looking for variety, you can change the speed and incline for all sorts of new challenges. And many of the fancy newer models feature programmed workouts for those days when you just want to be told what to do. On the downside, the treadmill is not going to be an ideal choice if your joints are feeling cranky and you're looking for something lower impact, or perhaps if you're tired and feeling less coordinated than usual. Even when treadmill mishaps don't hurt, they can be a tad mortifying. (Don't ask me how I know that, either.)

Elliptical trainers are a good low-impact alternative. They don't offer quite as much variety in their programming as treadmills, but you can alter the grade and resistance level to switch up your workouts. You can also change your pace and level of exertion by moving faster or slower. They do require a little getting used to if you're not naturally coordinated, but once you're familiar with the motion, it's easy and painless to hop on and get going.

Stationary and recumbent bikes require a little more setup. You'll need to adjust the seat and handles to suit your body, which will make the workout safer, more comfortable, and more effective. Once you're in place, though, you have the option of letting your mind drift in a way that you can't risk on equipment that requires you to play an active role in not falling down. There are even some types of indoor cycling training that actively encourage meditation exercises on the bike, so if you're feeling it, you can close your eyes and try some mindfulness work while you pedal. As long as you don't fall off the seat or collapse over the handles, you're good.

Rowing machines are another good choice for wandering minds. If you're not the most body-aware person on the planet, there might be a steep learning curve, because the movement takes a little practice—it's a challenging exercise, and it also takes some coordination to get all your limbs working together properly. But once you've got the rhythm down, the only things you'll have to worry about are keeping it going and breathing.

WHAT TO LISTEN TO AT THE GYM

Looking for something to entertain you while you work out? Here's how to figure out the best choices for your mood.

THE SOUNDTRACK

When you're into the workout but could use some background noise

- Comfort TV reruns you've seen a million times
- Movie scores
- Meditation apps

THE COSTAR

When you feel OK but need a push to keep you going

- Favorite songs
- Chatty podcasts about light or semiserious topics
- TV shows you'd watch while dicking around on your phone

THE HARDCORE DISTRACTION

When you need to focus on something—anything—other than your workout and the inside of your head

- Audiobooks
- Podcasts that focus on topics you're deeply into
- TV shows you've been waiting to see

The random bits—which might include VersaClimbers, air bikes, Jacobs Ladders, or old-school stair machines—are good for novelty. They're all different enough from the more commonly available options to give your body and brain something new to do. Most of them are also intense enough to be a useful source of distraction, if that's what you're looking for in your workout. They're definitely not what you need when you want to zone out but great for when you need a task to yank you out of your head and force you to focus on something else.

If your gym has a pool and you feel comfortable using it, you can also factor that into the equation. Swimming is also a great workout/distraction combo. So is deep-water running.

Beyond availability, your choice of cardio methods or equipment can come down to personal preference. So I suggest you try them all, like a kid plowing through a toy store. Your goal is to find a type of exercise that you enjoy or tolerate, so there's no need to get bogged down in anything that doesn't serve that end. Don't worry about what machine will ostensibly give you the "best" workout—the best workout is still the one you'll do. Don't pay attention to the awful calorie trackers on the machines and wonder if a different one will give you a better total. The numbers on those things are speculative fiction, anyway. Just go play. You can try one at a time for a longer workout, or do a sampler of a few minutes on each type of machine—whatever feels the most casual and the least intimidating. Have fun with the process and then think about which part was the most fun. (Or which part was the least un-fun.)

If your gym offers classes and you're comfortable with working out in a group fitness setting, I suggest giving any cardio-focused classes that intrigue you a whirl, too. You never know what might end up clicking. If something doesn't end up working out, you never have to go back. And if it *really* doesn't work for you, you also have the option of leaving the class before it's finished. You can politely excuse yourself. Or just quietly leave. I promise you that the vast majority of instructors will not think you're a terrible person or hold this against you forever. (In fact, there's a good chance they'll be grateful that you came at all. Group classes need to produce numbers to continue, which means that instructors need people to be registered for their classes to keep their jobs. By showing up, you boosted their attendance count—regardless of whether you stayed for the whole thing.) If the very thought of this extra dose of human interaction and potential awkwardness turns you off, you can also look into virtual group class options.

It's also worth finding out if your gym has heavy or free-standing bags for individual use. Boxing and kickboxing rounds on the bag are a fun and cathartic form of cardio. For extra motivation, you can imagine your target is the physical manifestation of whatever brain stuff is ailing you.

CARDIO ON THE STREET

Of course, you don't have to do your cardio in a gym. One of the best benefits of this type of training is how relatively easily you can take it outside. (It's not that you can't do mobility or strength training in the great outdoors, but it takes a little more planning and creativity. With cardio, you can just grab your gear and go.) This option is obviously wonderful for people who like being outside. But it's also useful for people who know being in the world is probably good for them, but can never find the motivation to actually go out there.

Sampling the real-life equivalent of cardio machines can be a lot more challenging than hopping from station to station at the gym. It's easy to run or walk outdoors—just put on supportive shoes and nonbinding clothes and get out there—but rowing, biking, and cross-country skiing (the inspiration for elliptical machines) all involve specific equipment and specific terrains. But you're probably familiar enough with most methods to know whether they will be fun and realistic. (Can't ride a bike? Probably not cycling. Nowhere near a river? Rowing won't be your outdoor sport.)

I suggest making a list of what might appeal to you and what feels possible for you. Go through the more obvious options like walking, running, and biking, but also think of what else might be possible. Inline or roller skating?

Skateboarding? Cross-country skiing or snowshoeing, weather permitting?

Once you've got your maybes, there is, unfortunately, one more factor you'll have to consider in our capitalist hellscape: cost. The "Have you tried exercise?" crowd loves to act like it's 100 percent free to do stuff outdoors. That's usually not how it plays out in reality. You don't have to pay a fee to use most outdoor spaces, but any equipment you'll need has a price.

This doesn't mean you're out of luck if you can't afford all new gear. There are ways to work around this issue, provided that you have the time and energy to put into searching. (It's also totally OK if thinking about this is too much for you and you want to skip to "Cardio at Home" on page 167, which has more affordable and easily accessible options. But before you go, may I interest you in a walk? That activity can be done with the shoes and gear you already own and it's great exercise.)

For the sake of trying things out, you can source gear from what you have lying around, what you can borrow cheaply (or for free), and what you can find in your budget. Wear a comfortable pair of all-purpose sneakers for your first walks and runs. See if you can borrow or rent other gear to test it out before you buy. Check out thrift shops, secondhand sporting goods shops, and classifieds to see what's available. You could even get ideas for workouts based on what you're able to find. My husband started a one-man rollerblading revival in the mid-2000s because he found a pair of inline skates for five dollars at a Goodwill.

Once you have an idea of what you might like and what you can make work, start playing around with your options. Focus on how the workout makes you feel and what you're getting out of it.

If and when something sticks, there are five things worth considering:

- Gear: If you want to do a specific type of cardio on the road, you will definitely want to invest in equipment that will fit your body and your goals. In most cases, it doesn't have to be top-of-the-line, egregiously expensive, or even purchased new. But you should get something that can be used for exercise and get it properly adjusted to fit you. The one thing you will need to shell out the bigger bucks for is running shoes, if you're planning to run. Ideally, you would be able to get to a running store, have your stride analyzed, and choose a pair based on that information. But not everyone has access to a good running store—and not everyone feels comfortable going into a store by and for Fitness People. If you would prefer to avoid these kinds of interactions, you can study the wear patterns on your other shoes to help determine which type of running shoe will best support you. (A quick online search for "running shoe wear pattern" will direct you to the resources you need to figure this out.) Running shoes are expensive, and they seem to be going up in price at a rate that far outpaces inflation. But they are a solid investment in injury prevention and comfort.

- **People:** Unless you live in the middle of nowhere, doing cardio outside means that other people will perceive you and potentially get in your way. You'll have to plan and navigate your workouts in a way that takes your comfort and everyone's safety into account. If your workout requires you to share space with cars, save it for times when you're feeling more alert. If you live in a densely populated area and you find crowds distracting or unnerving, you might want to look beyond sidewalks and roads. Parks and cemeteries are good options. School tracks that allow outside users after hours are another good choice for runners. (Some might permit cycling and rollerblading on the track, too, but it's best to check before you take anything other than your feet on their grounds.)

- **Routes:** After you get outside, you have to go somewhere. The biggest factors that should go into your route planning are safety and comfort. Once those are covered, though, you can start designing routes based on your goals and personality. If you're not feeling 100 percent energetic or you'd like to break your workout into pieces and see how it goes, stay close to where you live. Draw out a small loop that you can repeat several times if you're up to it, but that will give you a tolerable trip back home if you need to cut it short. If you know you'll quit as soon as it feels possible and you want to remove that temptation, plan a route that goes straight out and back. That way you'll have no choice but to put in that distance to get back home. You can also use destinations as motivation and run to a place or person you want to visit. One of my favorite workouts for one of my favorite clients was walking to Dairy Queen and back.

- Growing pains: **Gym cardio equipment like treadmills, ellipticals, rowing machines, and stationary bikes will give you an amazing workout, but these machines don't perfectly re-create the experience of walking, running, skiing, rowing, or cycling in the outside world. That doesn't mean they're better or worse, it just means they're slightly different to use. So if you switch between machines and outdoor exercises, you might notice that one feels weird or takes a while to get used to compared to the other. That's totally normal.**

If all of this seems like a lot to juggle, don't underestimate the value of throwing planning to the wind and just going for a #*%$ walk for your #*%$ mental health. I don't know if you knew this, but I think walking is amazing. A totally underrated form of exercise. Do not underestimate this all-time classic. It gets you outside. It gets your heart rate up. (And it can really get the blood pumping if you want it to. Have you ever tried speed walking?) It clears your head. It 1,000 percent counts.

CARDIO AT HOME

If you can't or don't want to take a single step off your property, there are also plenty of cardio-oriented things you can do at home. You won't have to worry about route planning or having an audience. As long as you're respectful of the other people who live in your general vicinity—e.g., not doing hardcore skipping routines at 3 a.m. if you have downstairs neighbors—you won't have to worry about planning your workouts around outside limitations like gym hours or daylight, either. You can even get weird if you want to. (During one dark period, the only kind of movement that remotely appealed to me was doing basic aerobics steps to Depeche Mode songs. You could argue that the impulse to do this came from not getting out into the world enough. But I wouldn't have been able to do the one workout I didn't hate without self-consciousness or judgment if I'd gone anywhere else.)

The biggest challenge with doing cardio at home is that you have much less space to work with. But there are a few ways you can get around that. One is to buy your own machine. I only recommend this option if you are *pumped* about the idea, or at least excited about what owning a machine can do for you in concrete terms. If indoor cycling is your favorite thing in the world and buying a bike will allow you to ride whenever and however you want, then it's a great choice. If you find yourself getting really into running but can't get outside at certain times or during certain seasons, then a treadmill will most likely be a solid investment. If it's something you think you *might* use or *should* use, it's not going to be worth it. I've seen people who bought strength equipment to force themselves to exercise develop a gruff fondness for the stuff. I have never seen this happen with big-ticket cardio gear. If you are wondering whether it's worth it, the answer is probably no.

Another option is smaller equipment. Get a jump rope and try a little interval training. Add some footwork drills if you want to get fancy. Buy an aerobic step and step on and off it at whatever speed you like while watching TV—or check out the impressive library of old-school step workout videos available on YouTube. They hold up surprisingly well. Pick up an agility ladder (a contraption made of nylon straps and plastic bars used for drills that are kind of like fancy hopscotch), clear a space on the floor, and play around with it. (If my own experience is anything to go by, this can also be a fun, low-pressure way for autistic people to work on their body awareness, because it involves patterns, repetition, and going at your own pace in a space where other people can't gawk or make fun of you.) If you've got the space and inclination, you could also consider a hanging or freestanding heavy bag. Punching and kicking things is one of the finest sources of cardio and stress relief in all of fitness.

Smaller equipment frees up a lot of literal space, but it also makes some mental space. When you don't have to worry about justifying a bigger ticket purchase, you'll be able to have more fun messing around and finding out what kind of cardio you like doing at home and when you like doing it.

It's also worth looking around your home or the vicinity for anything that you can use for your exercise. Do you have stairs, or a step or two, in your place? Is there a stairwell in your building that you could use for recreational purposes? That'll give you a hell of a cardio challenge. Do you have access to a pool for swimming or deep-water running? (I realize that's a long shot, but I'm currently in a 1970s building with a pool that is clearly a holdover from when it was a swankier address. There's never anyone down there and I've been having a grand old time splashing around and calling it exercise.)

Finally, you can adapt your workout to your space. Not everything will make a smooth transition from the streets to the sheets. If you run in place for half an hour straight, your calves will take forever to forgive you. But there are all sorts of smaller-range movements you can do to get your heart rate up that can be assembled and disassembled in the way we discussed in Chapter 4. Such as smaller bursts of jogging in place, maybe with your knees up for an extra challenge. Or doing bear crawls forward and backward in place. Or jumping jacks, mountain climbers, shadowboxing, fast footwork drills, and the aforementioned arm waving and cardio decrying. And there's always flailing around in bed for those days when you don't want to get out of it.

HOW HARD SHOULD YOU GO?

The answer to this question depends on how you're asking it.

If you really mean "ugh, how hard do I *have* to go?" then the answer is "maybe a little harder than you'd rather, but definitely not as hard as you

BUST THIS MYTH:
RUNNER'S HIGH

The runner's high is real, but it's misunderstood and extremely over-hyped. Some people do experience a brief euphoric rush during intense or long bouts of cardiovascular exercise. It happened to me once! But it doesn't work for every runner and it definitely doesn't kick in every time you go out.

If you've never felt a runner's high and are wondering if you're doing something wrong, the truth is that we have no real clue. We used to think it was a burst of endorphins, but that's been debunked. Now experts think it might have something to do with endocannabinoids, a type of neurotransmitter. My pet theory based on my own experience is that it's a desperate delusion. Whatever it is, it appears to be kind of a fluke. It's perfectly normal to feel anything but high during and after a run. (Also, keep in mind we're talking about a "high" as described by serious runners, many of whom are abstemious in other ways. It's like bodybuilders talking about a really good protein powder—it might be the best thing they've tasted in ages, but they're comparing it to plain chicken breasts, not chocolate.)

Besides, when I think back on my best runs, I don't reflect on those few blissful seconds. I think about the runs that stopped me from completely spiraling. Or the times the sun was shining just right and my favorite running song started blasting through my headphones. Those are the moments I run for. Mercifully, they're not nearly so rare.

fear." You want to challenge yourself, whatever that means for you today (and some days almost anything is going to feel challenging). But you don't have to work to the point of being sweaty, flushed, and jelly legged. Aerobic literally means "with oxygen," so anything that makes you gasp for air or makes your muscles burn with lactic acid buildup isn't aerobic exercise, anyway. And if you're exercising to feel better, there's no point in making yourself suffer.

You really don't have to suffer to get a mental health boost, either. The best level of effort for improving both your mental health and your cardiovascular fitness is moderate. If you want to think in terms of heart rate zones, you're looking at somewhere between 50 percent and 70 percent of your maximum heart rate (MHR), sometimes known as the lower-intensity and temperate zones. You don't have to calculate your max (or even current) heart rate for these, either; you can use the talk test. In the lower-intensity zone, you'll be able to comfortably carry on a conversation or sing. When you get into the temperate zone, you should still be able to talk, but not sing. If you can't squeak out more than a few words, it's probably time to dial it back a bit.

Once you've put in a few weeks of regular cardio workouts in these zones, you can start to consider whether you want to start challenging yourself with more intense efforts. But you don't *have* to. You can continue to do all your physical activity in these zones and still enjoy plenty of physical and mental health benefits.

If you do want to push yourself harder, though, the question becomes "How hard *can* I go?" When you have firmly established a base level of cardiovascular fitness and you have an actual desire to do so, you can push into the higher end of your aerobic capacity—and maybe even beyond that if you're doing high-intensity interval training. Unless you are intimately familiar with your body, how it ticks, and what it feels like when you make it do things, I don't recommend relying on your perceived exertion or the talk test for figuring out those heart-rate-training zones. Instead, do some research on heart rate training. Calculate your MHR and what percentages of it are good for your current training goals, get a heart rate monitor, and follow the numbers.

This is vital for your health and useful for getting to know your body better. As someone with chronic anxiety, I spent a lot of time with my heart racing in my throat. So I thought of that speed as a resting heart rate and thought I was absolutely terrible at cardio because I struggled when I got too far above it. I was shocked when I actually started measuring my efforts and learning what different training zones felt like. What I was considering a moderate aerobic effort turned out to be dangerously close to my MHR.

If you have an inclination toward self-flagellation or self-harm, you will also need to be honest with yourself about why you might want to push harder in a cardio workout. Are you doing it because you enjoy the feeling of doing the exercise or because you enjoy challenging yourself in that manner? Or are you doing it to punish yourself, make amends for something you did (or ate), or because you think that suffering and pain is what you deserve? If it's the latter, you'll need to either slow down or pick a different exercise for as long as you're in that headspace.

WHAT NEXT?

You can keep doing the same cardio workouts at the same level of effort forever if you want. Whereas progression in strength training is linear, and there comes a time in most workouts when you'll need to change up your routine to keep your muscles and mind engaged, progress in cardio is a little more fluid. There are a couple of different ways you *can* make your workout more challenging, but there's no pressing need to do so.

If repetition works for you—if the only thing getting you out the door is the desire to listen to your audiobook while putting your walking legs on autopilot, for instance, or if you just want to do that one *Sweatin' to the Oldies* tape you've memorized so you know exactly what to expect—then by all means, repeat. There's no hypothetical benefit to a "harder" workout that will outweigh the sense of routine, comfort, and accomplishment you get from your thing. My only suggestion is to add a little cross-training to your exercise regimen. Doing the *exact* same movements in the *exact* same way for a long period could lead to muscular imbalances and a higher risk of chronic overuse injuries. An alternate exercise that moves your body in different ways can help even things out a little, which can keep you generally feeling better and able to keep doing your preferred activity for longer. (If you love running, for example, look for exercise that gets you to move sideways and backward.)

If you have specific fitness goals or you're looking for something new, you'll want to do one of the following: either increase the level of effort you're putting into your workouts, or increase the time or distance you're doing them for. Over the long term you can up both of these aspects, but focusing on one at a time will be significantly better for your health and performance. Then incrementally add a little more to your workouts each week or so. Slow and steady really does win the race.

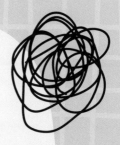

THROWING IN THE TOWEL

Deciding when to take a break,
skip a day, or quit

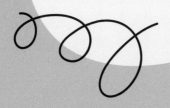

n my mid-twenties, I got it into my head that I should do mixed martial arts, so I signed up for a trial Brazilian jiu-jitsu (BJJ) class. It was slightly terrifying but exhilarating. I warmed up, sprinted, and attempted various animal walks and somersaults with the regulars. Then the instructors took me and another newbie to the small-scale octagon (the fenced-in ring used in mixed martial arts competition) in the back of the dojo, shut us inside, and gave us our first fighting lesson.

The skill I learned in the cage that day was the foundation for everything I did in martial arts. None of the takedowns, submissions, sweeps, head kicks, or combos I gave and received in the years to come would have been possible without it.

So what did I learn that was so bloody important?

How to give up.

In BJJ, when you know you're beaten or you're just ready for the fight to end, you tap. The actual act of tapping is quite simple. You repeatedly slap your hand against your opponent, signaling to them that you give up, and then they stop and let go. If your hands aren't free, you can say "tap" or otherwise verbally submit. We picked it up in a matter of seconds.

But then our instructor got into the philosophy and strategy of giving up. Say your opponent traps you in an arm bar, a move that puts their entire body and all the power their hips can generate against the stability of your elbow when it's being bent in the wrong direction. If they haven't applied the submission properly or locked it in just yet, and you know what you're doing, you can try to counter or defend. But if they've got your arm fully extended and they're starting to extend their hips to place more pressure on the joint, your elbow is not going to win that fight. At that point, it's over. If you can't recognize the moment right away, you might tap too late and end up with a sore elbow. You might miss a couple of days, and you definitely won't enjoy your next few training sessions. If you know it's over but your pride won't let you tap, you could end up with a broken arm and widespread soft tissue damage. You won't be doing any kind of exercise, let alone fighting again, for quite some time.

But if you know the warning signs and you accept them, you can tap, reset, and keep going. You can even take what you learned from your minor L and apply it to your next sparring session.

Not every sensei teaches this lesson well, or even believes it themselves. Not every student takes it to heart. And martial arts have their own problems, as far as their various relationship with bodies and society's hangups about them. But one major advantage that many martial arts disciplines have over general fitness culture is how matter-of-factly they approach the act of *stopping*: knowing and accepting when it's time, and moving on with as little self-reproach as possible. It's just part of the core curriculum and part of life.

This is the number one thing I took from my time at the dojo. I applied it to my work as a trainer, and I continue to use it in my own routines. And any time I feel my resolve slipping and I start to question whether I'm doing enough or giving up too easily, I remind myself that I learned this lesson in a fighting cage, and anything you learn in that setting has to be at least a little tough. Therefore, resting is tough and cool.

YOU DESERVE TO TAKE A REST

"You have to do this thing for your physical well-being" is an excellent lesson. But it's only a part of the greater rest picture. There's another lesson that is equally if not more important, and it's much harder for a lot of us to take to heart: you *deserve* rest.

There's a good chance you're struggling with this concept. Maybe you're thinking that the part about physically needing to take a break seemed convincing, but you were still feeling guilty about it for some reason. Or maybe you thought it sounded good for other people, but obviously this couldn't possibly work for *you*. (That's my brain's favorite response.) But it's true. Not only do you need to rest for your physical and mental health, you deserve to do this thing that will help you take care of yourself.

You deserve days where you don't have to do or think about exercise at all. You deserve to relax after a workout well done (or just plain old done, if you're being too hard on yourself to consider it good). You deserve to stop in the middle of a workout if it's hurting you or otherwise not going well for you. You deserve to relax and recuperate before you try again another day. You deserve to take a scheduled workout off your plate when you're feeling tired or overwhelmed. You deserve the relieved rush that comes from canceling a plan.

You're a human being, and you deserve to do a basic thing that is necessary for your mental well-being. For your very survival.

YOU. DESERVE. TO. TAKE. A. REST.

Seriously.

We need time off from physical activity almost as much as we need to sleep.

Sleep deprivation is torture.

DO NOT LITERALLY TORTURE YOURSELF.

BUST THIS MYTH:
"NO PAIN, NO GAIN"

I've made it clear how I feel about this concept from a physical perspective. But it's also used to encourage and glorify psychological suffering, so let's take a moment to reflect on how that's even worse.

Mental health isn't muscle fiber. If something makes a bunch of tiny tears in it, there's absolutely no guarantee that they'll heal, let alone grow back stronger. You're just as likely to end up even more exhausted and demoralized. (And even if it could make you stronger, why one earth should anyone *have* to suffer to experience the good things in life?)

Something else worth keeping in mind is that this slogan and many of its cohorts originated in the 1980s and were often geared toward a middle- to upper-class clientele. It flourished in a time of relative prosperity amongst people with some degree of comfort in their lives. There's a very good chance that the pain and exhaustion they were celebrating as their end goal is the starting line for many of us today.

If mental anguish and pushing yourself to your absolute limit and beyond actually did lead to gains, we'd all be jacked and thriving right now.

REST IS HARD, THOUGH

If you're still struggling to accept this—or you think it sounds good in theory but you've already come up with multiple counterarguments about why it couldn't possibly apply to you—you're not alone.

There are a number of reasons why it can be excruciatingly difficult to accept that you deserve to rest, let alone embrace it. I'm listing them in point form for easy access in case you need to return to them to remind yourself or anyone else. (If I can't convince you to rest right now, the least I can do is make your ongoing efforts to learn this lesson less mentally taxing.)

- **The world keeps telling us rest is bad.** Once you age out of your "go the f*ck to sleep" years, most people discourage you from resting at all. Directly and indirectly, we're told that we need to work hard and train hard. And somehow we're supposed to play hard in the few free seconds we might have at the end of the day. We're told rest is bad. Lazy. Selfish. Boring. You'd have to be superhuman to tune it all out.

- **When we are encouraged to rest, it doesn't look like rest anymore.** Rich white people have distorted and exploited the concept of self-care to the point that it either sounds like a full-time job or you'd need two full-time jobs to be able to afford it.

- **Once you get going, you might want to keep going.** This is particularly true if it's taken you a long time to find a form of physical activity that works for you and settle into a routine. If you're relieved it finally clicked, you may not want to stop. That's great, mostly! But see above, about rest being physically necessary, even if you're hyped.

- **Fitness culture gives us some really messed-up messages about consistency.** This is yet another case where fitness culture takes something that is true, blows it out of proportion, and ends up hurting the people it should be helping. When fitness pros and enthusiasts act like there's no point to working hard if you can't stay 100 percent consistent, far too many people become afraid that taking any time off will ruin all of their hard work. (Consistency is important in workouts. Or, I should say, it's important *when you can manage it.* You probably will find it easier to build and maintain the things you want from your workouts—whether that's strength, speed, stamina, jacked muscles, or a slightly unfucked brain—if you are able to do them on a somewhat regular basis. But that does not mean that random workouts will do nothing for you. And it definitely doesn't mean that taking necessary breaks makes you inconsistent, or that you'll lose everything if you rest. Guess what will mess up everything you've been working for, though? Not resting enough!)

- **You might be afraid of what comes after the rest.** If you didn't have the easiest time getting started with exercise, you might be worried that it will be hard to start again if you take a break. And you may feel you have to make up for the time you "lost" when you were struggling before.

- **If inertia made it hard for you to start, that same inertia can also make it harder for you to stop.** Maybe you can't stop. If your brain wiring doesn't love transitions and change, learning to switch between a state of rest and a state of activity can be a challenge.

HOWEVER, YOU STILL NEED TO DO IT

If you still can't convince yourself that you are worthy of rest right now, let's try a different approach.

You *have* to.

For the sake of your physical and mental health—the very things you're exercising for!—you need to rest.

Here are some consequences of not taking enough rest.

- **No refrain, no gain.** Exercise taxes the body. Rest is how it recovers and gets stronger. I went over this in Chapter 6, but it can't be repeated enough. Working your muscles creates little tears in your muscle fibers. When you rest, your body repairs these tears. That regrowth is what makes your muscles bigger and stronger. Exercising without resting is like cutting a sprig off a plant and expecting it to grow without planting it, watering it, or exposing it to sunlight.

- **Going without rest can be really, really bad for you.** Exercising too much without proper recovery can lead to overtraining syndrome. Symptoms of overtraining include loss of appetite, pain, fatigue, brain fog, weight fluctuations, lack of motivation, disturbed sleep, illness, and mood changes. In other words, doing too much can make everything that you wanted to improve worse.

- **It will make you feel bad in your body.** Even if you don't push yourself to the point of bona fide overtraining syndrome, training without resting will still put you at a higher risk of injury. The injury itself will suck. The amount of time you'll have to take off and the amount of effort you might have to put into healing and rebuilding will be the insult added to it. Even if you don't get injured, you could still end up way more tired and sore than necessary.

- **It will make you feel bad in your brain.** If you're overworked and sore and tired, what do you think that's going to do for your mood?

- **You could die.** For my fellow hypochondriacs: this outcome is rare and happens in extreme cases of overtraining. The kind of training we're talking about in this book is highly, highly unlikely to lead to death. Even if you're overdoing it. But if this is the shock you need to take care of yourself, then by all means keep it in the back of your mind.

REST 101

Once you accept that you deserve and need to rest, you have to learn how. In a perfect world, this would be instinctual. Your body would tell you it was ready for a break, and you'd recognize the signs and be able to respond in a way that would make it un-tired and ready to go again. But in a world that makes you question whether you even deserve a little break, you're probably going to struggle with the details.

The following guidelines can help you figure out what rest means for you. They're not hard-and-fast rules, and you're free to adapt them when they no longer meet your needs. But they'll do a good job of keeping you from destroying yourself while you learn more about your limits and how comfortable you are pushing them.

TAKE AT LEAST ONE REST DAY PER WEEK

At least one day a week where you don't even have to *think* about exercise. Some fitness experts will substitute "rest" with "reduced activity." They're not wrong, but this one depends entirely on the individual. If you're completely pumped about exercise, then doing light activity on your off days will be all-around good for you. If you have a relationship with physical activity any more complicated than that, though, I believe it will be far more beneficial for your mental well-being to give yourself some space from it. That doesn't mean that you can't do anything. If a friend invites you to go out for a walk, you don't have to turn them down because the lady from the book said you have to stay home. But you will absolutely benefit from having regular days or longer periods in your life where your body and brain can recover. In fact, the more resistant you are to this idea, the more important it is for you to commit to a regular rest day right from the beginning, and be serious about taking it. (And if you wind up doing anything that would not fall under "reduced activity," like a spontaneous high intensity interval training session, you will need to schedule a makeup rest day ASAP.)

ADAPT, RESCHEDULE, OR CANCEL WHEN YOU NEED TO

Do this anytime you need to—such as if you're too tired or sore to work out—as often as you need to. Yes, it's useful to follow some kind of routine in your exercise. Yes, consistency in your workout schedule will help you feel better consistently (instead of just while the endorphins are flowing). Yes, if you have to take significant time off for fatigue or illness, you may not get back up to speed instantly, and you'll need to learn how to tell when you're dangerously tired and when you're just out of practice. But the occasional surprise rest day or backup plan isn't going to sabotage all of your hard work.

If you are bailing on workouts so often that you can't establish any semblance of routine, that could be a sign that your current exercise plans aren't right for you. If you simply cannot bring yourself to face your workouts on a regular basis, it's time to start looking for something you'll dread less. If you're always too tired to exercise, then you might want to consider a less taxing type of workout (or a different schedule—we tend to think of early-morning exercise as more virtuous, but that's baloney, and if it's wrecking your sleep schedule to attempt early-bird exercise you should try working out at noon, or six p.m., or midnight). If you're too exhausted or in too much pain to get moving, then maybe exercise isn't what you need right now.

STOP WHEN IT HURTS

Discomfort can be a normal part of exercise. Pain is not. And while annoying fitness sloganeering will try to tell you that pain is temporary and a sign of weakness leaving your body, the truth is that pain is a sign that something is wrong. And if you don't pay attention to pain, that something could turn into a long-term issue that interferes with your goals and quality of life.

That includes mental and emotional pain.

If you feel something sharp and sudden while you're working out, stop and check on it. If something that's been feeling not great but manageable gets worse, check that out too. If you puke, definitely stop! Some fitness types still insist on glamorizing pushing yourself to the point of vomiting, but this is a sign that your body is in acute distress. Nothing good will come from continuing as you were once you hit any of these points. There's a good chance it will make things worse.

DON'T EXERCISE WHEN YOU'RE SICK

Before COVID-19, the general rule for exercise was that if your symptoms were all above the shoulders, you were probably good to keep going, but anything in the chest or lower was a sign you should rest. In the past couple of years, though, I've chosen to err on the side of caution and take time off regardless of where my symptoms are located, and I don't feel like that's caused me to lose anything or regress in my training. The choice is yours, but if you're looking for permission to rest when you're under the weather, here it is.

HOW DO YOU KNOW
WHEN IT'S TIME TO REST?

I can't provide solid answers to this question, let alone anything I can condense into handy points. Figuring out what your body needs and figuring out how to provide it is a lifelong process, and the world we live in is constantly mucking up that process.

When I was already years into my work as a fitness professional, I heard a fellow instructor say "listen to your body" during a class. I thought this was a revelation and immediately started using it in almost everything I did.

This might be my biggest regret about my career.

I'm not upset that I encouraged people to pay attention to what was going on in their bodies and to respect it. That's a genuinely good thing. But I wish I had been more aware that the suggestion was a first step, not a solution. I wish the way I employed it had been more respectful of how hard it is to actually do.

Most of us spend our entire existence being encouraged to ignore our bodies, to push them beyond what they can handle in every aspect of our lives, and to hate them. Listening is wonderful, but first you have to learn your body's language. You have to learn to pay attention to what is happening and what it feels like. Then you have to learn what those things mean. Then you have to learn what responses to those signals are healthy for you and how to respond without guilt or self-reproach.

None of that will instantly snap into place because a trainer encouraged you to do it. No matter how well-meaning and earnest they are.

Learning to communicate with your body is far from impossible, but it takes a lot of time and constant effort. When you make an honest attempt to pay attention to how you feel when you move your body in different ways, you'll learn the difference between the burn you feel in your muscles during your last couple of reps and the pain you feel if you tweak something during a lift. You'll learn what your breathing does when you're in the right cardio zone versus when you've been pushed outside it. And you'll start to figure out when to continue, when to reset, and when to stop. You'll get a sense of the difference between pushing yourself and punishing yourself. You'll probably spend the rest of your life working on the doing-it-without-guilt part, but there will be moments when things click into place.

So now, instead of telling you to listen to your body, I encourage you to start developing a rapport with it. And to be gentle while you're doing it. Especially in the early stages.

If you think you might need to stop, stop. If you're not sure whether some-

LESSER-KNOWN MEDALS YOU DESERVE

Professional, amateur, and recreational athletes can pick up shiny prizes for winning competitions and reaching milestones. Place in a bodybuilding tournament: you get a trophy. Complete a 5K run: you get a medal. If you win the right grappling match, they might give you a sword.

These achievements are all worth acknowledging, but they're not the only things worth celebrating. It's popular to mock "participation trophies," but whatever—a lot of achievements short of taking the gold, including wholehearted participation, count as wins in my book (and this is my book). Here are some other major accomplishments worth rewarding yourself for:

- Got out of bed.
- Finished a workout and felt good about yourself.
- Didn't finish a workout and still felt good about yourself.
- Didn't quite start a workout because you couldn't handle it, but got your sneakers on and got out the door.
- Didn't start a workout at all, because you knew you needed time off to avoid or heal an injury.
- Complained about exercise very creatively and entertainingly.
- Got through a cardio or weight workout in the gym without feeling bad that others were lifting heavier or running faster.
- Stood at the front of the group exercise class instead of hiding in the back.

thing is worth resting over, rest. If you find yourself pushing beyond what your limit might be out of some misguided effort to prove your worth—which is my depression's preferred way of screwing up exercise—then back off. If you're afraid that you're not pushing yourself hard enough or that you're cheating, keep this in mind: you're trying to discover the line between *enough* and *too much* in a society that tells us nothing is ever enough. Most people have internalized that message, and for a lot of us, our brains double down on it when we're in distress. If you're even entertaining the thought that you're pushing yourself too hard during a workout or that you might need a break, there's a good chance that you're really overdoing it.

And while you're at it . . .

GIVE YOURSELF SOME CREDIT

Yes, this is in addition to the credit I told you to give yourself way back in Chapter 1. Give yourself credit generally, but also, give yourself credit for every specific thing you accomplish, even if it doesn't seem like something people cheer for. What's the worst that can happen? You briefly feel "too" good about yourself? You're 188 pages deep into a book that's encouraging you to be kinder to yourself for the sake of your physical and mental health. I don't think you're at particularly high risk for a raging ego or complete lack of accountability or anything.

Congratulate yourself for a completed workout. Celebrate the parts of an incomplete workout that you did manage. Don't beat yourself up for a workout that you missed or skipped. Tough love is probably the last thing you need at a time like this.

I genuinely don't believe I'm going too easy on anyone when I say this. As a depressed personal trainer, I've done weight training, plyometrics, mixed martial arts training, and running. I once taught six cycling classes in a week on top of all that other training. I've done every sort of burpee workout you could think of. I once broke my toe during the warm-up for a Brazilian jiu-jitsu competition, rolled around on the floor wailing like Gollum, got up, and competed. (Which I don't recommend.)

And nothing has ever left me as physically and mentally drained as the simple act of staying alive. So if you're reading this, you're already doing the hardest workout imaginable. If you want to, when you want to, there's still time to figure out the rest.

You're doing a great job.

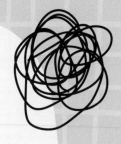

APPENDIX

Tracking your workouts and
staying motivated

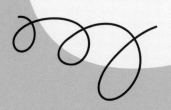

And we're done! Great work. Give yourself a big hand.

If this book were a fitness class, this appendix would be sticking around the gym to squeeze in a few more reps of something else you wanted to do before hitting the locker room. You have completed the thing and you don't need to do any more. So if you want to be done now, or you hate charts, thanks for coming! Stop reading now.

If you're feeling sufficiently encouraged to exercise but could use a touch more guidance on how to track what you're doing and stay motivated, the resources in the pages that follow can help. You might want to log your workouts because you find it motivating to know where you've been and where you're going. Or because you'll forget everything if you don't write it down. Whatever your reason, I've outlined four motivational styles that can help you decide how you want to set up a log, and samples for what each motivational style's ideal tracker might look like (the sample logs start on page 200). Where you keep that log—bullet journal, notes app, random scraps of paper strewn across your desk—is up to you.

This kind of classification, which is supposedly intended to help you toward greater self-understanding, always makes me feel paradoxically defiant. If you put me in a box, I'll break out of the box! If you put a boundary around me, I'll eat the boundary and wash it down with a cup of steaming-hot rules! When it comes to workout logs, though, I think it is useful to have a defined training style in mind that the log is tailored to. (And if you're the type of person who wants to use logs, you will probably be OK with that. You're here in the appendix, after all!) I've named the four types after the kind of tracking and motivation you're looking for as opposed to the type of exerciser you are, because I believe this is a more useful approach for our goals and because it made me feel less like I was writing a fitness magazine quiz in the 2000s.

If you've been paying attention to all of the places in the book where I said "if you [*like/feel/do things a certain way*] this might appeal to you because [*reasons this relates to your preferences/needs/goals*]," and you had a sense of which feelings and goals resonated with you, you might already know which style works for you. If not, I've included a flowchart on page 194 to help you figure it out.

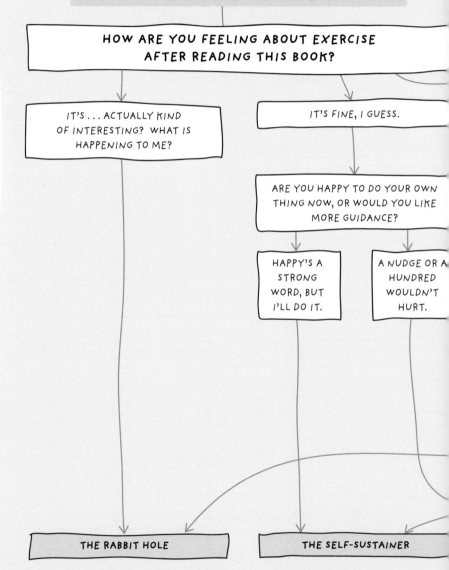

WHAT IS YOUR MOTIVATION STYLE?

HOW ARE YOU FEELING ABOUT EXERCISE
AFTER READING THIS BOOK?

IT'S . . . ACTUALLY KIND
OF INTERESTING? WHAT IS
HAPPENING TO ME?

IT'S FINE, I GUESS.

ARE YOU HAPPY TO DO YOUR OWN
THING NOW, OR WOULD YOU LIKE
MORE GUIDANCE?

HAPPY'S A
STRONG
WORD, BUT
I'LL DO IT.

A NUDGE OR A
HUNDRED
WOULDN'T
HURT.

THE RABBIT HOLE

THE SELF-SUSTAINER

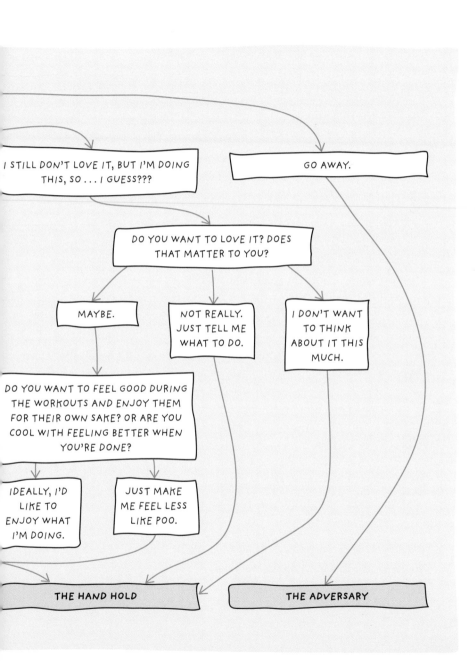

THE RABBIT HOLE

Once you got started, you realized you were kind of into this whole exercise thing. Not in the way a naturally talented athlete takes to gym class, but in the way the freshly hyperfixated dive into a new interest. You want to learn how the human body works and why—and what that feels like in your own body. And you want to figure out how exercise affects how your body works, why it works, and what it feels like when you're making it work. You might start getting weird cravings for anatomy textbooks and fitness manuals.

YOUR LOG

I've spent most of my fitness life in this style, and the type of log that I loved the most was an old-school running one that my mom gave me. While most of the other fitness templates were primarily numbers based, this one had a whole column dedicated to notes about the weather, heart rate, mood, or anything else you wanted to add. So you could keep track of the hard data but also keep an eye on how the entire experience was working out for you from day to day and week to week. When you set up your log, make sure to leave yourself plenty of space for data, research plans, and goals—but don't forget to pay attention to how you feel, not just to what you want to learn or achieve.

YOUR FITSPO

Instead of focusing on body types or athletic achievements, think about what you want your relationship to fitness to be like, and look for inspiration from people who embody that. My current exercise role models are a couple of professional wrestlers: Tetsuya Endo, for his excellent weight-lifting form and how thoughtful he is about his workouts, and Miu Watanabe, for her impressive strength and the gleeful enthusiasm with which she cultivates it.

THE SELF-SUSTAINER

Your relationship to fitness is neutral. You'll probably never love it, but it's fine. Whatever. You're perfectly content to do it as long as it helps you feel better. You have no problem with increased strength or endurance, but what you're really looking for is a feedback loop in which exercise makes you feel better, which makes you feel good enough to exercise, and so on.

YOUR LOG

This template has a similar approach to the Rabbit Hole, but with all of the nerdy bits removed. What's left is a chart that encourages you to focus on what you're doing and how that's making you feel in your body and your brain. It's detailed enough to give you a medium- and long-term overview of what's working and what isn't, but not so intense that it forces you to spend more time or effort on it than you want to.

YOUR FITSPO

Look for role models in people who use exercise as a tool to support something they're actually passionate about. Like a singer who runs to improve their lung capacity, or a grandparent who lifts weights so they can play with their grandkids a little easier. Or don't look for anyone at all, because that's more thought than you want to put into your routine.

THE HAND HOLD

You'll do the thing. Most of the time. But you won't *love* it. And your motivation isn't exactly what you'd call high. Or existent.

Exercise will probably always be a bit of a struggle for you, but you like the results when you do it, and you're willing to work for them. You just need an extra boost to help you get going. And then another one to help you keep going. And then maybe another one to help you get going again.

YOUR LOG

In the far left column, write down every exercise you might do over the course of the next week. (I've gone ahead and put rest in the first slot because it counts and is nonnegotiable.) The units can be as big or small as you want or need them to be. You can make the warm-up one spot, or give each move or minute of your warm-up its own line. You can even break each rep into its own line: "1 push-up," "1 squat," etc. After filling out the column, you're going to buy a bunch of cheap packs of stickers. Give yourself a sticker every time you do one exercise—put it right under the day when you did it. Set a goal for a certain number of stickers, and when you hit it, give yourself a little something as a treat that you define in advance. (This idea is very loosely based on my favorite academic initiative, the Pizza Hut Book It! program.)

YOUR FITSPO

Look for inspiration from people—or animals—who eventually got their shit done. Possibly through determination. Possibly through grumbling acceptance. Whatever speaks to you. If you're in a cheesy mood, you could always go with the tortoise from "The Tortoise and the Hare." If you're not, there's every single person and pet who made a "going for a stupid walk for my stupid mental health" video. Or the late, great Debbie Reynolds, who spent most of her 1983 workout video *Do It Debbie's Way* talking about how other home-exercise tapes were too fast, how little she was enjoying herself, and how she wouldn't have to do any of this if she'd had a hit record. Or the late, great Shelley Winters, who rolled around in the background of that video while gossiping about Howard Hughes and asking "are your bulges supposed to hurt?" (Clips are available online. It's worth a google.)

THE ADVERSARY

You are motivated by spite. You will do the thing, but you might swear about it under your breath and you will not have the demeanor of anyone who has ever appeared in a workout video while doing it. (Except for maybe Shelley Winters.)

YOUR LOG

You don't need your own log. You're probably getting annoyed at the very idea of one. You can pick one of the above and draw cartoon dicks on it, or something . . . and maybe fill in the parts that are useful for you and ignore the rest while you're there.

YOUR FITSPO

Think of every obnoxious gym teacher, coach, peer, parent, etc., who said you'd never get anywhere with that attitude. They're not the boss of where you get!

THE RABBIT HOLE

DAY	WORKOUT	THE HARD DATA (times, reps, sets, etc.)
MONDAY		
TUESDAY		
WEDNESDAY		
THURSDAY		
FRIDAY		
SATURDAY		
SUNDAY		

NOTES
(mood, observations, etc.)

THINGS I WANT TO
RESEARCH FURTHER

THE SELF-SUSTAINER

DAY	WORKOUT	HOW IS YOUR BODY FEELING?
MONDAY		
TUESDAY		
WEDNESDAY		
THURSDAY		
FRIDAY		
SATURDAY		
SUNDAY		

HOW IS YOUR BRAIN FEELING?	NOTES

THE HAND HOLD

EXERCISE	MONDAY	TUESDAY	WEDNESDAY
REST			

_____ POINTS UNTIL NEXT REWARD

THURSDAY	FRIDAY	SATURDAY	SUNDAY

NEXT REWARD IS _____

FURTHER RESOURCES

Here's a small list of other fitness professionals you can check out for tips, guidance, and workouts to get you started.

DEMI ADANNA

@fitgyal_demi on Instagram

There are many things to appreciate about Adanna's fitness account, which is filled with fun and effective exercises and helpful workout suggestions. But the number one reason I'm recommending it here is her brilliant Shy Girl Editions. This series of videos offers workouts that you can do in one place or with one piece of equipment. This means you can train at the gym without having to worry about taking up too much space, moving around from machine to machine, or socializing with others.

ROZ "THE DIVA" MAYS

rozthediva.com, @rozthediva on Instagram

Mays is an internationally acclaimed body-positive pole dancing instructor and personal trainer who has described her ideal clients as "plus-size athletes, gym virgins, and other misfits." Her content on Instagram (and beyond) is every bit as good as you'd expect from that description.

KRISTA SCOTT-DIXON

stumptuous.com

Scott-Dixon's website was like a bible to everyone I knew who was looking for BS-free information about weight training and related issues in the 2000s, and it holds up well. This is a good place to go if you're looking for exercise tips and perspective on the pursuit of fitness from someone who doesn't suck. And who wrote a book in 2012 called *Fuck Calories*.

SHERRI SPELIC

edifiedlistener.blog, @edifiedlistener on Twitter

Spelic is an author and educator from Austria whose work I appreciate for many reasons, but the reason I'm recommending her here is her work in physical education. Reading her insights is a must for anyone who wants to help someone else learn how to do stuff with their bodies in a not-awful way—and for anyone who needs to know that there are teachers out there who are doing good work and making the whole exercise thing better for the next generation.

EXERCISE PRESCRIPTION ON THE INTERNET

ExRx.net

I can't vouch for every single component of Exercise Prescription on the Internet. (I don't love that there's a weight loss section, for one.) But the exercise library, kinesiology section, and fitness calculator are all good, practical tools that you can use to learn more about how and why your body works and what you can do with it, without too much extra noise or nonsense.

ACKNOWLEDGMENTS

I'd like to take a moment to acknowledge the good influences I had in fitness in person: Giselle from Eclipse, who randomly took me under her wing one day. You probably shouldn't have been giving quite so many tips to a random member who wasn't paying for personal training sessions, but I hope I've made good on what you invested in me. Lhara Eben and Jane Clapp for opportunities and the guidance. And the excellent classes. Evan Boris a.k.a. Striking Concepts for being as good at coaching as you are at being a friend. Which says quite a lot. And Karen from STOTT Pilates for being the first instructor trainer I ever had who treated mental health like a component of our clients' well-being and not a marketing tool or something that could be forced into submission with the right moves.

While I'm here, I might as well shout out the good role models I've watched from afar: Trish Stratus. Jane Fonda. Richard Simmons. Georges St-Pierre and Erik Owings. Miu Watanabe. Tetsuya Endo.

On the writing side of things I can't thank the following people enough: My agent Stephanie Sinclair. Jane Morley and Kassie Andreadis for the precise and thoughtful copy edits. Elissa Flanigan for the amazing cover and interior design. And Jess Zimmerman for the idea, for thinking I was the right person to write it, and for being an absolutely brilliant editor. You made me like writing again. (Or like it as much as any writer can.)

And on a personal note, I'd like to thank the following for their all of their support and love: Aaron. Mom and Dad. My friends and family. And my assistant/coach Arcadia.